615.53

KU-267-543

ANGLO-

enemies
within & without

For V. L. Meek and E. P. Waters

We are a profession small in numbers but potentially unlimited in patient numbers and impact. All chiropractors know this but action to develop this potential is hampered by an external antagonist, the medical profession, and internally by ourselves.

('Information on JCC Activities', Joint Chiropractic Committee (New South Wales Branches of the United Chiropractors' Association of Australasia and the Australian Chiropractors' Association) 28 May 1985)

The enemy out there, if there's an enemy, it's us!

(Comment by a Queensland chiropractor, 1990)

ANGLO-EUROPEAN COLLEGE OF CHIROPRACTIC

enemies
within & without

Educating Chiropractors, Osteopaths
and Traditional Acupuncturists

Arthur O'Neill

La Trobe University Press
1994

First published in 1994 by
La Trobe University Press
La Trobe University
Bundoora Victoria Australia

Copyright © Arthur O'Neill

Typeset and printed by Aristoc Offset, Melbourne
Idea for cover by Sarah O'Neill
Finished art by Icon Art, Richmond, Victoria

National Library of Australia
Cataloguing-in-Publication data:

O'Neill, Arthur
enemies within & without

Bibliography
ISBN 1 86324 413 1

1. Chiropractors. 2. Chiropractic – Study and teaching. 3. Osteopathic
physicians. 4. Osteopathic medicine – Study and teaching.
5. Acupuncturists. 6. Acupuncture – Study and teaching. I Title.

615.53

All rights reserved. Apart from any dealing for the purpose of private
study, research, criticism or review, as permitted under the Copyright
Act, no part may be reproduced by any process without written
permission. Enquiries should be made to the publisher.

CONTENTS

ANGLO-EUROPEAN COLLEGE OF CHIROPRACTIC

ABBREVIATIONS

AAcA Australian Acupuncture Association – one of the occupational associations, mainly with members in the state of Queensland

AAC Australian Acupuncture College Incorporated – the Melbourne college considered in this study; commenced as a branch of Acupuncture Colleges (Australia) in 1975 when it was called Victorian Acupuncture Colleges (Australia). Incorporated as a non-profit making association in 1987

AC(A) Acupuncture Colleges (Australia) – founded in Sydney in 1969 and later with branches in Melbourne, Brisbane and elsewhere; still the name of the Sydney college and also used by the now separate Brisbane college

ACA Australian Chiropractors' Association – founded in 1938 to represent north American trained chiropractors; one of the two main occupational associations, merged nationally with the UCA in 1990 to form CAA(N)

ACATCME Australian Council on Acupuncture and Traditional Chinese Medical Education – educational standards and course accrediting body formed in 1989 by AESO

ACA(V) Victorian Branch of the Australian Chiropractors' Association

ACCE Australasian Council of Chiropractic Education – educational standards and course accrediting body

formed by ACA in 1974 and incorporated in 1977

ACCOE Australasian Council of Chiropractic and Osteopathic Education – 1990 modification of ACCE to cover osteopathy

AESO Acupuncture Ethics and Standards Organisation – a practitioner accrediting body closely associated with the Sydney and Melbourne acupuncture colleges (AC(A) and AAC)

AMA Australian Medical Association – the main occupational association

AMA(V) Victorian Branch of the AMA

AMAS Australian Medical Acupuncture Society – an association of registered medical practitioners of acupuncture

ANTA Australian Natural Therapists' Association – one of the two main alternative medicine associations (the other being ATMS)

AOA Australian Osteopathic Association – one of the two main occupational associations (the other being UOPG)

APA Australian Physiotherapy Association – the occupational association

ATMS Australian Traditional Medicine Society – one of the two main alternative medicine associations (the other being ANTA)

BSO British School of Osteopathy – the first school (1917) founded in the U.K.

CAA(N) Chiropractors' Association of Australia

(National) — the national association, formed in 1990 by the amalgamation of the ACA and UCA

CAAPIT   Chiropractic Alumni Association of Phillip Institute of Technology — the graduate association

CAE   Colleges of Advanced Education — a system of government funded tertiary institutions

CCA   Chiropractic College of Australasia — a Victorian college sponsored by the UCA which ceased operation on the 1978 incorporation of Victorian UCA members in the ACA

CSA   Chiropractic Society of Australia — an association of chiropractors, founded in 1985

DCSH   Department of Community Services and Health — the federal government department responsible for the NH&MRC

ICC   International College of Chiropractic — a private Victorian college sponsored by the ACA; its courses transferred to the PIT school of chiropractic but still exists as a professional continuing education body.

LI   Lincoln Institute of Health Sciences — a Victorian college of advanced education, later (1988) to become a school of La Trobe University

NH&MRC   National Health and Medical Research Council — a federal research funding body with state government representation

PIT   Phillip Institute of Technology (formerly Preston Institute of Technology) — a

Victorian college of advanced education

RMIT   Royal Melbourne Institute of Technology — a Victorian college of advanced education

SCC   Sydney College of Chiropractic — a New South Wales college sponsored by the UCA; from 1990 associated with Macquarie University

SCO   The Phillip Institute School of Chiropractic and Osteopathy — originally the private ICC; called the school of chiropractic from the 1981 inception of government funding; and with osteopathy added to the school name in 1988

SOT/SOTO   Sacro Occipital Technique/Sacro Occipital Technique Organisation — a chiropractic technique system and the association of its practitioners

TCM   Traditional Chinese Medicine

UOPG   United Osteopathic Physicians Guild — one of the two main occupational associations (the other being AOA)

UCA   United Chiropractors Association — one of the two main occupational associations; joined federally with ACA in 1990 to form CAA(N)

VIC   Victoria Institute of Colleges — a statutory body with constituent advanced education colleges, now defunct

VPSEC   Victorian Post Secondary Education Commission — a state government co-ordinating authority

INTRODUCTION

This work concerns the education of three small groups of alternative health workers: at the School of Chiropractic and Osteopathy, part of the government-supported Phillip Institute of Technology; and at the Australian Acupuncture College, a private operation run by an incorporated non-profit making association. Both teaching institutions are located in Melbourne. Since the study was conducted, Phillip has become part of the Royal Melbourne Institute of Technology (formerly a college of advanced education but now re-minted as a university); and the acupuncturists have succeeded in getting a degree programme started at another new institution — the Victoria University of Technology — made out of the combination of former advanced education colleges in western Melbourne.

Chiropractic and osteopathy began in nineteenth century America. Teaching commenced in 1892 in Kirksville, Missouri (osteopathy) and in 1898 in Davenport, Iowa (chiropractic). A few graduates from these and other American schools practised in Australia from around 1909 (osteopathy) and 1919 (chiropractic). Private Australian colleges started to offer chiropractic and osteopathy education in the 1920s but often in combination and also in association with other alternatives like naturopathy and homeopathy. Their graduates shared in the denunciation of orthodox medicine and the advocacy of nature cures but overseas-trained practitioners repudiated them. Chiropractic and osteopathy had each been announced as the whole of medicine. They were not only held to be quite different from each other but also from all other medical theories and practices. American osteopaths had taken on surgery by the time chiropractic began and later (after much division) they added drug therapy. This consolidated the gap between osteopaths and chiropractors. However, in Australia and the United Kingdom medical practice was strictly confined and overseas trained osteopaths were unable to utilise these techniques. Until the 1940s only a few American-trained osteopaths (and not many more chiropractors) practised in Australia. Some were prosecuted, usually for calling themselves doctors, which was against the law.

The numbers of overseas trained chiropractors and locally trained manipulators (who preferred the osteopath title) began to increase in the 1950s. After early success in Western Australia, the statutory regulation of chiropractic spread to all the Australian States and Territories following the report of a federal committee of inquiry (Webb, 1977). The registration of osteopaths was also supported by the committee and some but not all jurisdictions make explicit provision for it. The committee's registration proposals were tied to the institution of a course of qualifying manipulative therapy instruction in the official system of Australian higher education.

The federal government started to fund an accredited undergraduate chiropractic programme at the Phillip Institute in 1981. An osteopathy course began at the same place in 1986 after also obtaining accreditation and funding. At the start of this study, the Phillip school had been graduating chiropractors for a decade and the first group of osteopathic students was completing the third year of the five-year course. The communal life of the occupations is informed by the achievement of registration and formal higher education despite strong opposition; and by the arrangements made for the teaching of both courses in the one place despite hereditary antagonisms.

Russell Jewell, a chiropractor, started Acupuncture Colleges (Australia) in Sydney in 1969. In 1973/74 he opened interstate branches, including one in Victoria. The Australian Acupuncture College in Melbourne became a separate operation but remained closely associated with the Sydney college. Each ran similar four year programmes of evening and weekend study. Many private colleges, off-shoots of Acupuncture Colleges (Australia) and others that were separately founded, have presented acupuncture alone or in combination with natural therapies. Their number has declined but the Melbourne and Sydney colleges competed with them. Other health workers — chiropractors, naturopaths, physiotherapists and registered medical practitioners — use acupuncture or apply electrical and laser stimulation and manual pressure on acupuncture points.

The traditional acupuncture educators associated with the Melbourne and Sydney colleges sought occupational registration and the incorporation of their courses in the higher education system. The chiropractors wanted to consolidate earlier gains by transferring to a university, obtaining hospital access for clinical education, extending the length of the undergraduate course, and improving research and postgraduate education opportunities. The osteopaths were likewise concerned, with added preoccupations that come from being the minor partner in a chiropractic school. Occupational associations shared these interests and extended them to other enhancement projects, such as obtaining patient fees reimbursements through the federal government's universal health insurance scheme. Chiropractors, osteopaths and traditional acupuncturists thus aspire to the privileges and benefits enjoyed by registered medical practitioners.

KEEPING OUT THE ALTERNATIVES

Many conventional or regular medical practitioners have no time for alternative theories and remedies. Yet there is no self-evident justification for dismissing them. If explanations are answers to questions then, as Flew says (1985, 40), there may be 'as many, not necessarily exclusive, alternative explanations as there are legitimate explanation-demanding questions to be asked'. What counts against the medical alternatives, however, is the presumed availability of a litmus test of validity. Science enables them to be judged and found wanting.

This verdict about therapies is carried over to their exponents. The problem with the alternatives, according to establishment wisdom, is that they and their practitioners are intrinsically unsound. Having failed to make the scientific grade, alternative medical practitioners are considered irrational. They are a social liability, contributing to the misfortune and sometimes even to the deaths of patients. Therefore it is proper to anathematise them, in the interests of public safety, and to keep them out of convivial range. The institutions of health care, in particular the hospitals, are unavailable to them. Enclosure and isolation are the lot of most alternative practitioners. A 'colour bar' is sustained by a collective belief in the existence of a distinction between those medical occupations that are scientifically informed and those that are not.

In this study I examine the consequences of segregation for students and teachers of chiropractic, osteopathy and traditional acupuncture. An added (and unexpected) ingredient is the antagonism of practitioners for each other. Leaders of alternative medical associations are always preaching unity in the face of established medical enmity. That they are impelled to do so evidences longstanding divisions within each occupation. This only solidifies the arguments of critics who maintain that treatment protocols and work standards are not kept up by fragmented organisations, and that the failure to unify them demonstrates the incoherence of practices and the absence of effective self-regulatory measures. Governments and their agencies have pressured alternative medical associations to settle their differences and merge as a preliminary to the enactment of practitioner registration and the introduction of tertiary education in officially supported institutions. But alignments and disputes cannot be considered without taking into account the imperial shadow cast over all the alternatives by medical orthodoxy: how alternative practitioners frame the distinctions that set them apart from other members of their occupations, as well as how they formulate their singularity and worth, are related aspects of the experience of continuing diminishment.

Foucault (1989, 65) speaks of attempting to understand society and civilisation 'in terms of its system of exclusion, of refusal, in terms of what it does not want, its limits, the way it is obliged to suppress a certain number of things . . . its repression-suppression system'. I consider the exclusion of certain health care occupations from the side of those who are being educated to join and those who teach in them. The aim, in short, is to pursue Max Weber's project of interpreting action in terms of its subjective meaning. That requires an understanding of the meaning of the work and the world for the students and teachers of chiropractic, osteopathy and traditional acupuncture. In conveying their interpretations I neither support nor deny what they have to say, but I do note that their conceptions of themselves as members of groups are bound to, and are incomprehensible without reference to those designated as internal and external occupational antagonists.

Most of the following chapters are episodic in character, each being devoted to an issue of moment that occurred during the term of my study. I use the particularities of disputes to leave a composite impression. A few remarks may serve to introduce general features. The three medicines are considered as social movements whose advocates seek to transform extant understandings of sickness and its alleviation. Some also want to make qualifying courses of instruction in the image of the education offered by university medical schools. This transformation from within is intended not only to demonstrate reputability but also to secure it. Such endeavours fail to satisfy external opponents and exacerbate internal tensions. At issue are conceptions of fitting place, relations with occupations in the same field, interpretations of historical mission and degrees of allowable variation from them. Struggles are often inconclusive but affiliations change in the course of them. Group regulation is tightened, at the cost of membership alienation and the exclusion of elements judged unacceptable. Conflicts over doctrine and strategy accompany the reproduction of organisational division. Some emphasise strict adherence to the distinctive messages of their medicines and seek to maintain clear lines of enclosure. Others stress complementary features of practice and wish to secure an integration (though not the amalgamation) of healing groups. Despite these basic differences, combats over principle and tactics are cross-grained by numerous pacts. The alliances are of a piece with the discords. One has to get inside the life of a group in order to discover the relational textures.

I spent two years in the company of students and teachers, attending classes, clinics, meetings, formal events — participating in the daily round — and talking in bars, cafeterias, restaurants and tearooms and I read at least some of the vast amount that has been written by and about their medicines in texts, tracts, journals and official correspondence. The custom is to refer to this way of going about other peoples' business as the method of participant observation and to claim scientific credentials for it. But a lesson I learnt from being amongst those condemned for their want of science was to doubt that Science offers a royal route to the ordering of experience. Observation and participation only are queer bedmates if one presumes a species difference. Besides, investigators can be so lost in the illusion of objectivity that they fail to recognise what the 'subjects' make of them. Towards the end of my stay as an engaged onlooker, I asked a final year chiropractic student what others thought of my regular presence in their clinic. She replied:

> You're the strange guy with a past that rings a bell of academia but now a student in the crowd who is hanging around the place and asking questions. No one knows why you are there and what your purpose is. But you're pretty harmless, and O.K.

My purpose is to transmit and to inform their experience. To that end, I was present and distant, a combination that is never secure and is always rich in ambiguities. The science of it, like the medicines, is compounded with art and philosophy.

An explanation of social life is more than a taxonomy of its features but the chaos of the material is, somehow, contrived into a form which conveys a partial version of what has been seen, heard and read. Dollard (1957: 369) speaks of the varying standpoint of the observer and classifier of incidents who moves in cautious circles around the complex event — in his case, the traditional order of Negro subjugation in the southern United States during the 1930s. This work also moves about an unending variety of possible interpretations — of the systematic diminution and isolation of chiropractors, osteopaths and traditional acupuncturists — without readily settling on any one.

I have not attributed the quoted statements of practitioners, students and teachers. They are left in a frequently expected and sometimes required anonymity. Fabricating names only makes sense if one has a manageable cast but mine was in the hundreds. Their words are drawn from my field notebooks. Leaders are impossible to disguise. Their opinions carried positional influence and I have identified them by title where that seemed relevant.

The details of internal papers, correspondence, statistical information and certain articles are given in chapter endnotes. The main sources are occupational newsletters, archival deposits and working files of the teaching institutions. The bibliography is confined to journal articles, monographs, official publications and theses.

I express my gratitude to the University of New England, which made a grant towards the publication of this book.

I

THE EDUCATION ESTATE

Here we are getting our diplomas. I guess that means we're professionals now!

(Speech on behalf of graduates, 1988 acupuncture graduation ceremony.)

INTRODUCING THE SCHOOLS

The Phillip Institute of Technology, one of the more recently established higher education institutions, used to hold its graduation ceremonies in the great hall of Victoria's oldest university, the University of Melbourne. The ceremonies were lengthy occasions, for the president of the Institute council handed out each testamur. To accommodate the press of numbers from the eight Institute schools, multiple events were held around May each year. There were three in 1989 and four in 1990.

Each ceremony followed a routine. Wilson Hall, a cream-brick, glass-sided rectilinear building replacing the 1882 Gothic original that burned down in 1952, was packed. The graduates in their academic robes were seated at the front. An organist played sombre music. The audience stood as a dignified processional tune ushered in the director of the Institute, members of its council, a guest speaker and a small but stalwart band of academic staff from the schools offering graduands that night. This company took up seats on the stage. The ceremony began with some choral music. One year there was J. S. Bach's *Nun danket Alle Gott* and Vivaldi's *Gloria* and the next a specially composed *Intrada*. After a few words from the college director, the presentation of awards and a convocation address, the stage party and the graduates retired to a celebratory toccata. They were bound for tea or coffee and cakes in the sparse student union banquet room.

They left behind some thirty-five chiropractic graduates who took over the stage for a rite of affirmation. The dean of the School of Chiropractic and Osteopathy told them they had joined a profession with tremendous career prospects and opportunities for self-actualisation:

> But remember your duty to do good. You are healing through the skill of your hands and the sharpness of your minds. May you be successful and good people. You have completed one of the most demanding courses in the higher education system.

A member of the profession administered the Chiropractic Oath, with the initiates following in plainchant:

> I do hereby affirm before God and these assembled witnesses that I will keep this oath and stipulation:

> To hold in esteem and respect those who taught me this chiropractic healing art; to follow the methods of treatment which according to my ability and judgment I consider for the benefit of my patients; to abstain from whatever is deleterious and mischievous; to stand ready at all times to serve humanity without distinction of race, creed or colour.

> With purity I will pass my life and practice my art; I will at all times consider the patients under my care as of supreme importance; I will not spare myself in rendering them the help which I have been taught to give by my alma mater; I will keep inviolate all things revealed to me as a doctor of chiropractic.

> While I continue to keep this oath unviolated, may it be granted to me to enjoy life and the practice of the chiropractic healing art, respected by all people at all times.

Bearing the ceremonious imprints of vanished institute and school control, these new-found Bachelors of Applied Science (Chiropractic) departed for their turn at the refreshments.

After photographs and the return of academic regalia ('an Oxford-style black undergraduate gown, and a silk-like hood with white edging'), many of them ended the evening at a local pub. They had been away from the school for nearly twelve months by the time each graduation ceremony came around but there was a firm group opinion: not to come back. 'Ours was the first year when they decided to start punishing students', says one, 'and I tell you what, I'm leaving the school with a bad taste in my mouth'. Another, a graduate from an earlier year, maintained that much the same happened when he was a student: 'I was glad to get the piece of paper and leave. Most go and don't want to see the school again'. He also said that the school was too scientific in its approach and was not sufficiently aware of what chiropractors needed and did:

> That's why the students want more philosophy. When you are in practice you try a whole variety of things. What you are trying to do is find something that is successful at getting the patient better. It's true others find it difficult to accept chiropractic when its techniques are not standardised, when a variety of methods are used without any consistency.

There was much critical talk about the shortcomings of 'the administration', 'the powers that be'. A third graduate asserted that he did not want to play the sort of games the school administration plays:

> There are people who never did the work who are graduating – one guy last year, for example, fabricated some of his cases. But he got away with it and he is graduating tonight while there are others who have been held back because they did not complete [the casework requirements].

They proceeded to talk about a trial arrangement where a few students have been allowed to take their residency programme in a South Australian hospital. These students told them how amazed medical doctors and students were to find out how much education and knowledge the chiropractors had; how they could read x-rays better than many medical interns; how they could rule up the x-rays and tell them what was there. The hospital internship was considered to be a breakthrough for chiropractic. It was very hard to get adequate clinical training unless students gained a much wider experience than the school could provide through its clinics. By the following year, the hospital had revoked the arrangement. Optimism was always being dashed but was forever kept up. Sometime, somehow, medical opponents would come to realise what patients already knew – that chiropractic was efficacious and chiropractors the members of a worthy and well-trained profession.

The inaugural graduation of chiropractors from this school took place a decade before. Twenty Australians, a New Zealander and a Swede (three women and nineteen men) received diplomas from the privately run International College of Chiropractic (ICC) in May 1979. The awards were 'approved' on the evening by Dr Barry Ritchie, the principal of what then was called the Preston Institute of Technology. Eighteen months later, in January 1982, Preston was to amalgamate with another advanced education college to form Phillip.

The first ceremony, conducted at Preston's Bundoora site where the International College was located, was in much the same form as the more recent ceremony. Those chiropractors who kept to their oath hoped to be granted the respect of all men rather than of all persons. Afterwards there was a dinner dance at La Trobe University, located a few kilometres away from Preston in the same outer north-eastern suburb of Melbourne.

Emeritus Professor Rod Andrew, a former dean of the Monash University medical school, was the occasional speaker at the first event. He told the audience that when he qualified in medicine over forty years before:

> Osteopathy and chiropractic, it would be fair to say, were regarded by orthodox medicine as an imposition on a gullible public, a form of cultism in the pejorative sense, if not downright quackery. The pre-Darwinian axiom *nulla species nova* — no new species — no new kind of doctor was contemplated.[1]

Andrew sketched his association with chiropractic. In 1967 he had been a member of a committee appointed by the Australian Medical Association (AMA), at the invitation of the Victorian government, to investigate and report on chiropractic and to advise whether it should have statutory recognition and be registered as a profession:

> We reported that the time was not yet ripe and I believe this was the correct decision then. However, we also stated that given the acceptance by the chiropractic profession of certain requirements, registration should be considered.

The conditions amounted to a specification of educational orthodoxy — a matriculation entrance standard, 'educational principles proper for a professional course directed to health care', proper evaluation and course accreditation — and an act of parliament setting up a registration board like the medical board. Andrew said these criteria had been met and exceeded. He had not the smallest doubt that as the International College 'becomes more and more integrated with and part of the total life of the Institute [it] will go from strength to strength'. Andrew told the graduates: 'You are increasingly becoming part of the team of professional first contact — While the team is ineluctably the core of health management, nonetheless all members have their own unique role'.

The ceremony marked a transitional stage for the International College as well as for the graduates. Such events are 'dramas of persuasion'; the ritual is 'an instance of high courtesy' (Myerhoff, 1977, 222). Andrew's speech comfortably linked occupational progress – a rational advance from cultism to membership of the health care team – with the efforts of his audience and in response to specifications laid down by the AMA. But Andrew later told a researcher:

> The AMA committee at the time thought they'd built enough walls and dug a deep enough ditch and filled that with enough bullshit to make it impossible for any chiropractic group ever to fulfill all those conditions (quoted in Willis, 1983, 181).

Rites of passage are systematically connected to the structure and adjustment of social relations as Gluckmann emphasises (1962, 4-7). Andrew did not so much paste over medical condemnations as propitiate absent furies. He delivered an oracle:

> I hope, I expect, that the Australian Medical Association will be animated by a generous and co-operative attitude towards your profession which now has amply demonstrated its unimpeachable standards of education and its unexceptionable statutory control through the Victorian Chiropractors Registration Board.

That did not jibe with experience or expectation but the artifice of graduation rituals is to construe previous and future events by the celebratory rules of amity and progression.

The AMA had just re-affirmed that it did not recognise any exclusive dogma such as homeopathy, osteopathy, chiropractic and naturopathy, and that: 'It is unethical for medical practitioners to associate professionally with the practitioners of such dogmas'.[2] Chiropractic might have become a registered occupation with a course of qualifying instruction in a higher education institution but over a decade later the divisions were, if anything, sharper. The prognostications of graduation speakers were belied by a fixity of official medical opinion about the alternatives.

The director of Phillip highlighted another transition in his 1990 opening remarks. He said:

> These are perhaps the last ceremonies conducted under the title Phillip Institute. The whole education scene is being changed by direction of the federal government . . . I guess there may be a little

sadness when the name Phillip Institute of Technology disappears but the Institute is moving to the university sector.

Nevertheless, Wilson Hall had been booked for the following year, just to be on the safe side.

The federal government wanted to increase higher education enrolments and to reduce the number of self-contained institutions. Most of the Victorian colleges of advanced education had been or were about to be absorbed by universities, or, in one instance to combine to form a new university. Phillip was in the middle of painful amalgamation negotiations with La Trobe University.

A year earlier, the director had been widely criticised by college academics for dragging his feet when he should have been pursuing a merger. The chiropractors were strongly in favour of incorporation. They had always wanted to belong to a university. Joining La Trobe (which did not have a medical faculty but had recently acquired a health sciences school) could only promote the recognition that was due to chiropractic.

There would be little change to the graduation ceremonies if an amalgamation occurred, save their removal from the inner-city University of Melbourne to neighbourly La Trobe. The acupuncturists hoped to have much more rearranging to do. The staff of the Australian Acupuncture College pursued government control of acupuncture practice through the registration of practitioners and also worked to have their private course transferred to a university (La Trobe was in their sights). Chiropractors had been in very much the same position over a decade earlier and the acupuncturists sought to follow their example.

The 1989 Australian Acupuncture College graduation was held on the upper floor of a Chinese restaurant in the city. The La Trobe Vice-Chancellor, one of the deputy vice-chancellors and the dean of the Health Sciences School were guests. The seating was carefully arranged to expose them to the cause. There were thirty graduands but only fifteen received their diplomas on the evening. The others departed shortly afterwards to undertake a clinical placement at the Beijing College of Traditional Chinese Medicine and they wanted to have their ceremony there.

The principal of the college gave a speech after the first course of the meal. He said these graduates were special for the staff. They were not only the largest but also the most diverse and enthusiastic group and they were entering the profession at a most exciting time, through the incorporation of acupuncture into its rightful place in the Australian health care system. He thanked La Trobe for providing them with expert tuition in the health sciences. His message was reinforced by the next speaker, the principal of the allied Sydney acupuncture college, which also was looking for admission to a university. The two colleges were, as the Melbourne principal told me later, 'working towards having two branches of the one college in different universities'. The Sydney principal stressed how keen she was to see acupuncture move into the recognised government tertiary education system. 'In New South Wales', she told her Melbourne audience, 'we have achieved the highest standards of training with government accreditation of our course. We have an accreditation application for a two year post-graduate diploma course for medical practitioners, physiotherapists, chiropractors and osteopaths to overcome the poor standards of training available to these groups'. She proceeded to confer the awards. One of the graduates brought the house down by coming forward in an academic gown. Other speakers then urged graduates to join the Acupuncture Ethics and Standards Organisation (AESO) and to participate in the affiliated Society of AESO Practitioners. The president of the society told them that it 'suffers from stagnant Qi [meaning a lack of energy or drive — see the next chapter for a discussion of the term]. Now you have graduated, give back some of your Qi to the profession!'

The Sydney college had held its ceremony a few months earlier, in a restaurant in the botanical gardens on a balmy summer evening. The first floor space merged with the trees and birds flitted around the edges of the audience. As happens on such occasions, the graduates were made into instances of institutional achievement — they were the first to get a 'recognised' award for their studies.[3] Speaking on behalf of the premier of New South Wales, a parliamentarian said it was an historic occasion, for this was the first and only government to have accredited an acupuncture qualification. The AESO president told the audience:

> I can remember a time when we could be regarded as quite sinister. There was a time when we thought we would be banned. This ceremony is a significant part of Australian history. Australian *acupuncture* history I mean!

Another speaker made one of those inversions which makes evident that modernity is the custom of a place:

I'm very pleased to see we have at last a fully accredited course. Non-traditional medicine has a lot to offer. If non-traditional medicine is to be able to get what it deserves ultimately it must be accepted by traditional medicine.

The organisers of both graduations were well pleased. After the Melbourne event, the La Trobe Vice-Chancellor was reported to have said that he would see acupuncture in the university before retiring at the end of the year. The health sciences dean had reassured college leaders that an extremely critical report on acupuncture brought down a few months earlier by Australian government's principal medical research funding body, the National Health and Medical Research Council (NH&MRC), would not affect the incorporation. To judge by the speeches at the Melbourne graduation and at the Sydney event a month earlier, traditional acupuncture was but an inch away from being registered and gaining university courses leading to practice qualifications in Sydney and Melbourne.

Some teachers and graduates were less content. One said that systematisation had its disadvantages:

When we started it was very hard. We only had one very inadequate room. There were diverse students, some without education, housewives, all sorts. But they could do it, they got through the course. All this is to go, to be made into a slipstream. There's a lot lost by formalising and regularising it.

But acupuncture colleges had been criticised for enrolling all sorts of students. Writing to the NH&MRC's Health Care Committee about the acupuncture inquiry it had agreed to establish, a Queensland medical practitioner and acupuncturist drew attention to the lowly employment and lack of educational prerequisites of students and staff in a nearby College of Natural Therapies.[4] He said that if acupuncturists were to be registered, a grandfather clause would be sought:

thus legitimating the already numerous 'clowns' dispensing acupuncture. Do we really want electricians, petrol pump attendants and upholsterers doing 3 day/week courses in half-baked colleges dispensing medical advice and opinions?

Chiropractors also could criticise the irregularity of students. One, recently returned from overseas education and so unknown locally, was sent to look at the course provided by a private college which his occupational association opposed. Over twenty years afterwards, he recollected 'It was full-blast stuff. There were housewives, bikies, people in sandals, people who were away with the pixies. It was full-on!'

A few days after the Melbourne acupuncture college graduation there were uncomfortable moments at an in-service seminar. The teachers had been discussing changes to the procedures for course assessment and five of the new graduates (who had been asked onto the staff) were invited to comment and to compare what was proposed with their experience as students. Their criticisms of former arrangements elicited explanations and justifications from the Melbourne and Sydney principals who interrupted to make them. The leaders were quick to defend and protect the course, even from their own. But they thought the weekend had been a success. Staff wanted further training and were moving into a new year in a new way by writing down their course outlines, objectives and assessment procedures. The course was to be 'made more professional' in order to have a smooth transition into La Trobe. One of the new staff said to the rest 'I'm going to form a union! I want fifty bucks [an hour] for this! The students will learn how to be mercenary after four years!'.

THE PROFESSIONS: SIZE, INCOMES, ATTITUDES

In mid-1990 there were 2 106 chiropractors and osteopaths in Australia.[5] The majority, 86%, were chiropractors, with 9% osteopaths and 5% either registered as both or registered as chiropractors in one state and as osteopaths in another. *Dynamic Chiropractic*, an American newspaper (whose by-line is 'Mailed every two weeks to every doctor of Chiropractic, chiropractic student and chiropractic supplier known to exist on the planet earth') was circulated to some 50 000 chiropractors.[6] The United States had by far the most practitioners (44 000). Canada came second and Australia third. Other countries were well behind. There were more chiropractors in Australia than in all the countries of Europe. The Australian contingent was quite significant in the world of chiropractic, not least because the Phillip school was the first (and for a long time the only one) to achieve a funded programme in a government-supported higher education institution. In 1990 the other Australian teaching institution — the Sydney College of Chiropractic — was incorporated in Macquarie University, and so joined Phillip in obtaining government backing.

Australian chiropractic was a male profession: only 16% of those registered in 1990 were women (up from 14% at the end of 1988). Osteopathy attracted rather more women (23% in 1990, up from 20% in 1988). Nearly all the practitioners ran private clinics or worked in them. A 1985 survey of a chiropractor sample found that 96.8% of the respondents were employed in this way, with 1.1% engaged in teaching/research and 1.4% in other activities (0.8% no response).[7] Chiropractic incomes are attractive. The survey (pp. 27-28) attempted a reconciliation of reported incomes and calculations derived from reported patient visits. The median reported gross annual income was $A62 000, with 32.5% of respondents earning $A90 000 or more and 36.4% earning $A49 000 or less. Patient-load calculations suggested considerably higher figures. However the authors of the survey reckoned these were probably overestimates since 'it is likely that chiropractors follow the medical pattern of taking one day or a half a day off through the week for recreational purposes'. In rough terms we can say that chiropractors earned about as much as self-employed medical practitioners, dentists and the like. Some earned a very great deal and others were in the middle to upper professional income bracket. Whether osteopaths did as well was quite unclear. By their own account, for approximately the same fee they spent much more time per visit with patients than did chiropractors. Thereby, osteopaths evidenced their greater worth, not their comparative wealth. You could make a healthy living in both occupations.

Compared to other primary contact healing occupations (i.e. ones that do not depend on patient referrals), chiropractic was small and osteopathy minute. There were six times as many registered Australian physiotherapists and seventeen times as many registered medical practitioners as there were chiropractors and osteopaths.[8] Relative sizes will scarcely alter. Chiropractic and osteopathy intakes, which stood at 120 in 1988, had not increased much over a decade and were expected to stay close to this figure. First enrolments in the ten Australian medical schools only slightly declined over the same period and were supposed to stabilise at around 1 400. Compared to physiotherapy, chiropractic and osteopathy have gone backwards: the five physiotherapy schools enjoyed considerable growth to 1989.[9]

Therapies overlap and there is, besides, the burgeoning trade in Sports Medicine. Spinal manipulation has been so taken up by physiotherapists that it forms a regular part of their activity. This occupation has a predominantly female workforce.[10] Only a quarter are in private practice whereas with the male physiotherapists it is exactly the reverse: three-quarters of them are in private practice. Thus, the sex composition of physiotherapy, chiropractic and osteopathy private practitioners is not so different: males compete with males for the 'bad back' business. A good number of registered medical practitioners also use manual techniques. A small sample survey of general practitioners (conducted for a Victorian parliamentary committee) found that 49% had personally used manipulative therapy in their practice and 25% would consider using it (87% had not used/would not consider using osteopathy/ chiropractic therapies).[11]

One can infer that a larger number of physiotherapists and registered medical practitioners utilise manipulation than there are chiropractors and osteopaths. Though the latter represent themselves as expert in manipulative *techniques* (with reason, having been extensively trained in them and using them as standard practice), the former do not have high opinions about chiropractic and osteopathic *therapies*. Physiotherapists are almost uniformly opposed to chiropractic (though they tend to keep mum about osteopathy – a few physiotherapists have also trained as osteopaths). The general practitioner sample made a distinction between the effectiveness (but not the potential harmfulness) of manipulation – which many of them used, though infrequently – and chiropractic/osteopathy therapies (only 15% had recommended that any of their patients go to chiropractors or osteopaths):

Table 1   General Practitioner Sample: Attitudes to Manipulation and Osteopathy/Chiropractic

	(%)			
	Highly effective	*Moderately effective*	*Seldom effective*	*Don't know/ no response*
Manipulation	17	65	14	6
Osteo/Chiro	7	48	35	10
(Dixon, 1986, 214; extracted from table 1)				
	Frequently harmful	*Occasionally harmful*	*Never harmful*	*Don't know/ no response*
Manipulation	13	82	1	4
Osteo/Chiro	12	76	2	10
(Dixon, 1986, 216; extracted from table 2)				

In summary, chiropractic and osteopathy are small, well-paid, predominantly male, private practice occupations. Manipulation, the occupational bread and butter, has become increasingly popular with the other main primary contact practitioners — physiotherapists and registered medical practitioners — who considerably outnumber chiropractors and osteopaths. In each direction (and also between chiropractors and osteopaths) distinctions are made about the effectiveness of therapeutic techniques. Manipulation — adjusting bony joints, particularly those of the spinal column — means different things to different groups. In addition, there are various massage, or soft tissue techniques which are employed conjunctively by most chiropractors and all osteopaths and physiotherapists.

Traditional Chinese medicine must have been widely used by the Chinese who came to Australia during the gold rushes of the mid-nineteenth century but there are few surviving records. In 1893, On Lee sought to have his conviction for using the title 'doctor' overturned.[12] He produced evidence that he was qualified in China, having studied for 12 years in a hospital in Canton and in another Chinese hospital for 12 years also. He produced his title to the rank of Mandarin of the 4th class. But he failed. The judge held that the law prevented any unregistered person from holding himself out to be a doctor of any kind.

On Lee seems to have come to attention for advertising in the Melbourne *Age*. Prosecutions are still mounted, at the instigation of state medical boards and after complaints from the Australian Medical Association, but the most recent have been unsuccessful.[13]

Asian immigrants brought indigenous medical practices with them and there are many practitioners to be found in Chinese and Vietnamese areas of the cities. But estimates of the numbers of traditional acupuncturists in Australia are scant. As noted earlier, many registered health professionals employ acupuncture, with 10% of general medical practitioners reported to have been using it in 1986-87[14] and 21% of the respondents to the 1986 Victorian parliamentary survey saying that they had personally used it in practice (Dixon, 1986, 218). Acupuncture might be an infrequent resort amongst these practitioners and the diagnostic methodology originally associated with it is unlikely to be utilised. By all accounts, the therapy is most often an adjunct and is used empirically (as a supplemental measure and for cases where experience or hearsay suggest the possibility of benefit, especially for pain relief). Rather the same holds for many of the unregistered practitioners. Like physiotherapists and general medical practitioners, many pick up acupuncture by way of short courses. Some naturopaths and other natural therapists obtain a little acupuncture training during their preparatory education. Acupuncture is a magnet that draws all manner of practitioners to it.

Though they did not know much about or think much of oriental diagnostic methods, the general medical practitioners in the Victorian survey considered that acupuncture was somewhat more effective and somewhat less dangerous than chiropractic and osteopathy (and more of them recommend patients go to acupuncturists — 67% versus 15%):

Table 2   General Practitioner Sample: Attitudes to Acupuncture/ Acupressure/Oriental Diagnosis

	(%)			
	Highly effective	*Moderately effective*	*Seldom effective*	*Don't know/ no response*
Acupuncture	13	62	23	2
Acupressure	1	28	36	35
Oriental diag method	3	3	34	61

(Dixon, 1986, 214; extracted from table 1)

	Frequently harmful	*Occasionally harmful*	*Never harmful*	*Don't know/ no response*
Acupuncture	2	77	14	6
Acupressure	2	25	36	37
Oriental diag method	5	13	15	67

(Dixon, 1986, 216; extracted from table 2)

In Australia, traditional acupuncture might be a career but more often it has been a sideline. Some trained in the traditional ways (in courses offering three or more years of education fully devoted to traditional Chinese medicine or solely to traditional acupuncture) were also qualified in other health occupations and continued in them. They did not necessarily go on to use acupuncture as a major element in their therapeutic work. One natural therapies organisation estimated there were 400 practitioners of traditional Chinese medicine in 1988.[15] The figure is related to practitioners giving 8 treatments per day for 4 days per week and so is an attempt to indicate those engaged full-time. A 1993 AESO survey, conducted through a journal which is not confined to members, garnered responses from 93 full-time practitioners.[16]

AESO itself (which began in alignment with the Sydney and Melbourne colleges and was rather selective) had 282 members in

1988 (and 323 in 1990, plus 40 associates who were accredited but not practising).[17] Women made up 39% of the membership in 1988 and 36% in 1990. Accreditation by this group was quite restricted and not all of those eligible joined it. Some of the members in acupuncture practice were also involved in other therapies and many only practised part-time. An AESO practitioner checked the 52 Victorian members in 1989 and found that only half were using acupuncture and only about a quarter were, in any sense, full-time.

Few people earn all or most of their living from traditional acupuncture and other Chinese medical practices — perhaps no more than the 400 mentioned above. But the situation could alter if acupuncture were to become a registered occupation, with many otherwise unregistered and potentially eligible practitioners switching appellations. This is what happened with chiropractic. In the prospect of its registration, many locally-trained manipulators ceased to use 'osteopath' or 'osteopath and chiropractor' titles and became plain chiropractors instead (Webb, 1977, 32).

Apart from a few highly visible self-promoters who are despised by the rest, few traditional acupuncturists appear to earn much from their work. The AESO practitioner mentioned earlier booked 3–4 patients an hour and considered this to be the limit. Also at least the equivalent of a day in the working week was taken off because the practitioner found the work was so intense. On this basis, gross income would be up to that for a middle-range chiropractor but it has to be stressed that the acupuncturist was amongst only a handful in Victoria who were considered by peers to be qualified for, and to have made a success of, full-time practice. Most only made pin-money from acupuncture.

Enrolments in acupuncture courses are falling. The peak year for the college studied here was 1988 when it had an intake of 34 and a total student body of 100. In 1990 the intake was 12 and the total (at mid-year) was 51.[18] Sydney college enrolments also had declined. Some other colleges have closed or are no longer accepting students in separate traditional acupuncture courses. The financial situation of most of these small private institutions is shaky. Getting registration and courses transferred to higher education is therefore something of a last-ditch stand to keep traditional acupuncture alive.

To sum up, acupuncture is not licensed anywhere in Australia. Its exponents are split between competing schools and professional associations and many of the exponents mix acupuncture with other therapeutic practices. Little information is available about numbers of practitioners and the range of their activities. Very few of those who call themselves traditional acupuncturists or practitioners of traditional Chinese medicine earn a full living from the work. With rare exceptions, their incomes from this source are quite low. Like manipulation, acupuncture is employed in other (mainly private practice) occupations like registered medicine, physiotherapy and, to a lesser extent, chiropractic.

The success of the alternatives is usually measured by increases in the numbers of practitioners and widespread public acceptance of their remedies. The Victorian parliamentary committee (Dixon, 1986, vol.1, 25-26) reported there had been exponential growth in the number of practitioners listed as acupuncturists, herbalists or homeopaths in the 'Yellow Pages' of the Melbourne telephone directory. The committee went on to say:

> After a fairly static period in the early 1970s the numbers of alternative practitioners trebled between 1975 and 1980 and again between 1980 and 1986. This growth has been most marked in the categories of naturopaths and acupuncturists, whereas listings for homeopaths and herbalists barely changed at all until the mid-1980s.

Surveys by the committee found that 22% of the Victorian population sample had used alternative medical practitioners (of naturopathy, homeopathy, herbalism, iridology and acupuncture) in the previous five years (Dixon, 1986, vol.2, 35).

Data, such as that in the Dixon report, is often presented by alternative practitioners as evidencing a spring rain of achievement and by the members of state-licensed or 'regular' medical occupations as a warning-signal of a flood of irrationality. This brief account indicates that chiropractors, osteopaths and traditional acupuncturists are far from being so significant a medical presence as they, and their opponents, represent them to be.

The Dixon committee information is, at any rate, unconvincing. According to a bar chart in the report (v.1, p. 26), the number of alternative practitioners advertising in the 'Yellow Pages' (they are not disaggregated) rose from around 50 in 1970 to around 550 in 1986. A perusal of the 1990 'Yellow Pages' acupuncture entry shows that a simple addition does not reveal the numbers of people practising acupuncture as such and there are two possibilities of multiple counting — from double entries under the one therapy and from the combination of entries under it and under other therapies. Chiropractors, naturopaths, and osteopaths offering this service are listed together with some medical practitioner clinics and physiotherapists. Some individuals have two entries – by name and under professional association listings. Further, any estimate is not meaningful without comparing it to the growth of other medical occupations. According to census figures, the number of Australian registered medical practitioners doubled between 1971 and 1986 (from 16 105 to 32 788).[19]

Finally, any calculation also must take comparative frequencies of consultation into account. The Dixon committee found wide variation amongst the 22% of Victorians who had visited alternative practitioners over the preceding five years – the average being three visits per year (1986, vol.2, 49). Information was not collected on the frequency of visits to orthodox practitioners or to chiropractors and osteopaths (who were not reviewed because they were already registered).

Alternative medicine enjoys considerable public support but what has spread, over some twenty years, is the adoption of acupuncture and manipulation by orthodox practitioners (though they rarely, if ever, endorse chiropractic, osteopathic and traditional Chinese theories). More patients are likely to discover these alternative therapies by being offered them when they go to physicians and physiotherapists than by patronising alternative practitioners.

THE TEACHING INSTITUTIONS

Nothing could better indicate the benefits of government support than a comparison of the facilities and staffing of the Phillip School of Chiropractic and Osteopathy and the Melbourne acupuncture college. The former occupies part of an eight-storey, stark red brick and concrete building originally designed to house an engineering school. An osteopathic clinic is also located in this building and there are three suburban chiropractic teaching clinics. A chiropractic and osteopathy clinic has since been built on the campus. There are the usual teaching laboratories, lecture theatres, a library and a student cafeteria but hardly any research space. The colleges of advanced education were supposed to be vocational institutions and they were not funded to undertake research. Two other Phillip Schools –

Applied Science, and Human Movement and Physical Education —
provide service courses in anatomy, biochemistry, biology, chemistry,
microbiology, pathology and physiology. Other Phillip staff also teach
small units in psychology, sociology, communications, statistics and
research methodology. The Bundoora campus of Phillip is largely
self-contained and located in extensive parklands. It is surrounded by
new housing estates. Many staff and students travel considerable
distances to get to it. By early evening the place is deserted.

Teachers complain about the facilities and the funding available
to the chiropractic and osteopathy school. It is the smallest of the
eight Phillip schools and that leads to concern about an internal
merger. Everybody might come together to complain about being
short-changed by government but there are tough school
competitions for space and money. Teachers in other schools
maintain that chiropractic and osteopathy are overfunded for the
numbers enrolled. The school resents the amount of 'its' funding that
goes to the service departments and, more particularly, their separate
existence. The leaders say that anatomy, microbiology and pathology,
for example, ought to be part of the school.

For all the complaints, the Bundoora campus is modern and
stands up well in comparison with other advanced education colleges
or former colleges. Still, Phillip is a bit of a shock to newcomers,
partly because of its remoteness from the city centre. One staff
member from overseas said that from all she had heard in
chiropractic circles about the great achievement of chiropractic in
getting into a reputable government-funded institution, she expected
Phillip to be what the University of Melbourne actually looked like.
They were kilometres and worlds apart. While Phillip had a nursing
school, a legacy of the placement of chiropractic and osteopathy
courses in the college was their educational separation from the two
university medical schools and from other therapy courses, most of
which were offered by the Lincoln School of Health Sciences which
had joined La Trobe University.

The acupuncture college rented a small, old former shop in an
established eastern suburb of Melbourne. Behind a reception room,
in which the college administrator and a secretary also worked, there
was a single clinic room. A rear extension had a tearoom, which led
onto the principal's office. Apart from an outside lavatory, that was
all.

At the start of 1989 there were 84 enrolled students and, in addition to the principal, eleven teachers.[20] 'Many of us are old hippies', the principal said. Some had come to acupuncture by way of their interest in eastern philosophies. Only a few had gone into acupuncture straight from school; most had undertaken tertiary courses and worked as teachers, nurses, or in other professional occupations.

Students attended lectures at the Lincoln school which rented rooms to the college each Sunday. Through one of its service departments, Lincoln also had contracted to provide anatomy, physiology and other subjects — called 'western medical sciences' by the acupuncturists — on a student fee-paying basis. These were offered on one evening per week. There were some evening acupuncture tutorials in addition (conducted in a rented room at an inner suburban education centre). In the later years, students went to private practitioner clinics to get up their 300 (subsequently changed to 400) clinic hour requirement. Sunday, when the teachers and students in all years were present at Lincoln, was the liveliest day at the college.

The college depended on tuition fees — around $A3 500 a year per student for the combination of acupuncture and western medical science subjects in 1989. Chiropractic and osteopathy students, like other students in universities and advanced education colleges, did not have to pay fees (though after many years of 'free' higher education, the federal government introduced a standard charge in 1989 to be paid on enrolment or collected as a tax after income reached a threshold). Higher education institutions and students were heavily subsidised by the government. Chiropractic and osteopathy students worked full-time at their studies, the exceptions usually being those few who were repeating failed subjects. Acupuncture students worked full-time to finance their evening and weekend study. Their college had next to nothing of its own. There were few complaints about facilities.

Like other private schools teaching alternative health courses, the acupuncture college was distant from official higher education. Even the association with Lincoln was slight, confined to some staff in one department, and with teaching conducted at times when other Lincoln staff and students were not present. The college made much of the connection, which evidenced support for its purposes. But there were Lincoln teachers who thought that traditional acupuncture was bunkum. Many in the Lincoln physiotherapy department (which offered acupuncture training to physiotherapy graduates) opposed the incorporation of the college.

SUMMARY

Here were small groups of people with brave intent and high aspiration. Chiropractors, osteopaths and traditional acupuncturists sought to have their importance recognised. They were sustained by convictions of rectitude that were derived from foundation teachings — the myths that are, according to Sorel (1961, 50), not descriptions of things but group expressions of a determination to act. But restrictions on access to the hospitals and other public health facilities, the separation of courses of study from university medical and allied therapy schools, and the orthodox repudiation of theories and healing claims all served to keep them isolated. Versions of their empirical practices had become part of the therapeutic stock of physiotherapists and registered medical practitioners, which only elevated the occupational barriers. Patient bodies were the battleground on which the sides contended.

NOTES

1. Andrew, R. 'Graduation is the end of the beginning', *Chiropractic College News* 5 (2), July 1979, p. 2. International College of Chiropractic.
2. 'Policy on relationships with other health professions', *Medical Journal of Australia*, Supplement 1 (5), 29 July 1978, p. 14. This proscription had been first enunciated in 1965, in response to the imminent proclamation of a West Australian Act regulating chiropractic, following an earlier Royal Commission to investigate a proposed Natural Therapists Bill which recommended chiropractic licensing (Guthrie, 1961). A federal assembly then resolved that: 'The Australian Medical Association is of the opinion that medical practitioners may not act in consultation with, associate professionally with, conduct investigations for, or refer patients to chiropractors or osteopaths'. 'Relations between the A.M.A. and Chiropractors', *Medical Journal of Australia*, Supplement 1 (17), 19 June 1965, pp. 126-127.
3. On the establishment of government funded advanced education colleges in the mid-1960s, a system to regulate awards was instituted. State certification bodies investigated and accredited advanced college (but not university) courses. Approved college and university awards were maintained on a federal register, a sort of stud book of Australian tertiary courses. The idea was to secure national standardisation, no easy matter when all things to do with education belonged constitutionally to the states and the tertiary institutions harked on their autonomy. The register was a means to conformity: having a registered award was a necessary (but not sufficient) condition for federal funding. A scheme of course levels was given expression by standardised nomenclature — associate diploma, diploma, undergraduate degree, etc. — related to admission requirements, years of study and course content. In some states (such as New South Wales) the accreditation of private college courses was allowed. The

Melbourne college also sought accreditation but the Victorian legislation was murky and over a year was wasted while the state co-ordinating authority sought legal advice before rejecting the possibility. On the Sydney acupuncture college certificate, the award — Diploma of Applied Science (Acupuncture) — was asterisked to a footnote legend: 'The Australian Council on Tertiary Awards National Register Certificate No. 4435'.

4. Strauss, S. 'A Brief Look at Non-Medical Acupuncture', Attachment to agenda for NH&MRC Health Care Committee, 16-17 September 1987, DCSH files.

5. Statistics are drawn from the *National Register of Chiropractors and Osteopaths* (July 1990) compiled by the Chiropractors Board of South Australia from state and territory registration board records. After allowing for multiple state registrations, the totals were: chiropractors — 1 783; osteopaths — 204; registered with joint titles or as chiropractors in one state and osteopaths in another — 119. The occupations were growing slowly: there only had been a net increase of 181 in overall registrations since the previous compilation in December 1988.

6. *Dynamic Chiropractic*, breakdown of circulation, 7, 2, 15 January 1989, p. 4.

7. *Report to the National Chiropractic Consultative Committee on a Review of Chiropractic Services - 1985.* Brisbane, University of Queensland/Uniquest Limited, September 1985, p. 20.

8. There is some variability in the estimates of registered medical practitioners and physiotherapists, which depend on factors such as: converting part-time employment to full-time equivalent; allowing for net migration; allowing for multiple State registrations; allowing for registered but inactive persons; reconciling data from various sources. For a discussion of the registered medical workforce, see Doherty (Chairman), *Australian Medical Education and Workforce into the 21st Century*, Canberra, Australian Government Publishing Service, 1988, pp. 365-512. The figure used here is the committee's adjusted workforce estimate of 34 415 medical practitioners as at June 1986 (p. 434). Various projections suggest slow increases in numbers to 44 000-48 000 between 1986-2021 but decreases in doctor:population ratios from somewhat under 1:440 in 1986 to around 1:470-510 in 2021 (pp. 436-437). The 1988 estimate for registered physiotherapists, 11 449, is a collation of State and Territory registrations by the Australian Physiotherapists Association: *A.P.A. Membership Data*, 5 September 1989.

9. The 1988 Phillip intake was 75 in chiropractic and 25 in osteopathy. A further 20 enrolled in the Sydney College of Chiropractic. Medical school enrolments and projections are from *Australian Medical Education and Workforce* [Ref. 8], p. 417. Physiotherapy enrolment figures come from the Australian Institute of Health's *Health Workforce Bulletin No. 27: Preparation of Health Professionals Through Tertiary Education in Australia 1989*, Canberra, Australian Government Publishing Service, 1991, pp. 16-17. There were 645 commencing undergraduate physiotherapy students (428 females and 217 males) in 1989. The subsequent addition of an undergraduate course (at the University of Melbourne medical school) and possibly a Masters course leading to first professional qualification (at Monash University in Melbourne) will widen the gap between numbers of completing physiotherapists and chiropractors/osteopaths.

10. No adequate national physiotherapy statistics are available. The summary here is drawn from *Physiotherapy Workforce Statistics Victoria: December 1987*, prepared for Physiotherapists Registration Board of Victoria by the Health and Workforce Planning Unit of the Health Department of Victoria, December 1988. Female respondents to a questionnaire of all Victorian registrants were 80% (table A14), 53.3% of them worked part-time (defined as up to 34 hrs. per

week), whereas 88.1% of the males worked full-time (table C1). After conversion to full-time equivalence (40 hrs. p.w.), 25.2% of the females and 73.9% of the males were in private practice (table C11).

11. Dixon, J. (Chairperson), *Inquiry into Alternative Medicine and the Health Food Industry*, Social Development Committee, Parliament of Victoria, December 1986, vol. 2, pp. 214, 216, 218, 221.

12. *The Australian Law Times*, vol. XV, 1893, pp. 42-43.

13. A Victorian magistrate held that a Beijing graduate in Chinese medicine 'did not pretend to be and use the title of Doctor of Medicine' within the meaning of the section of the Medical Practitioners Act which prohibits unregistered persons from calling themselves doctors of medicine. Power, P. *Summary of Proceedings*, Detective Senior Constable I.M. Andrew and Liu Dan, in the Magistrate's Court at Prahran, 18 May 1992. The AMA said that it considered Power's findings and comments were 'baffling': 'How the Magistrate could be satisfied that Mrs Liu Dan was not pretending to be doctor of medicine when she was claiming to be a "specialist" in the areas mentioned totally mystifies us. [She said she was a specialist in Gynaecology, Paediatricology, Otolaryngology, and Orthopaedics in a letterboxed pamphlet.] In our opinion the Magistrate's decision certainly does not reflect the intention of the Act and we do not intend to let the matter rest. Perhaps it's a case of not only alternative medicine but alternative law'. 'Magistrate rules Chinese herbalist is a Doctor', Australian Medical Association, *Victorian Branch News*, June 1992, p. 102.

An acupuncturist of Sri Lankan birth (a qualified medical practitioner in that country also holding a Ph.D in acupuncture) was summonsed in Western Australia for contravening the Medical Act by holding himself out as being willing to perform a medical service and by using the title of doctor. He was found not guilty on the first count. While guilty on the second, the magistrate used his power to dismiss the case. The medical board has lodged an appeal to the Supreme Court. See the reports and comments in Resnick (1993, 63) and Berle (1993, 64).

14. Minutes, NH&MRC Working Party on Acupuncture, 15 October 1987, DCSH files. The estimate, based on rebate claims under the national health insurance scheme, counts practitioner deliveries of one or more acupuncture treatments over 1986-1987 (more recent Health Insurance Commission records indicate 3 003 medical providers of acupuncture in 1990/91 and 2 947 in 1991/92). The working party reported (Westerman, 1989, 68) that there were in excess of 2 800 provider numbers, that is, medical practitioners who were registered to provide rebatable services under Medicare and whose patients actually claimed rebates for acupuncture services. The working party was unable to distinguish general practitioners from specialists but it would be reasonable to suppose the majority were general practitioners. This suggests that 15-20% of these practitioners delivered acupuncture, though the DCSH records indicated that some did so infrequently.

15. *A case for the Registration in Australia of Naturopathy, Traditional Chinese Medicine (Acupuncture), Remedial Therapy*, April 1989, S. VI. 3. 2., Australian Natural Therapists Association.

16. 'Results of the A.E.S.O. Inc. questionnaire', Acupuncture Ethics and Standards Organisation memo, 30 March 1993.

17. AESO membership records as at 10 October 1988 and 12 October 1990.

18. Australian Acupuncture College records as at 17 July 1990.

19. *Australian Medical Education and Workforce* [Ref. 8], p. 413.

20. The staff list showed a Director of Studies, 3 Senior Lecturers and 7 Lecturers. All were casual (paid by the hour) employees and some had only a few hours of teaching association with the college each year. Only three were practising

acupuncture in anything approaching a full-time way. Four were school teachers; one an advanced education college lecturer in a business school; one ran a veterinary practice; one was employed as a microbiologist; and one had a pension.

II

THE MESSAGE

The Chiropractic system, revised on earth today,
Was known in ancient ages, in regions far away.
Sages and seers proclaimed it of origin Divine
And practiced it in secret, at many a hollowed shrine.

The great, new light that's breaking o'er all the widespread earth,
Is calling mystic knowledge to wider, further birth.
So, 'mid the great revival of truth among mankind,
This truth, contained in Nature, must wide acceptance find.

(W.J. Colville, in D.D. Palmer *The Chiropractor's Adjuster,* 1910, 21)

INTRODUCTION

Dissident systems of medicine flourished during the nineteenth century, especially in the United States. Osteopathy, and then chiropractic, were relative latecomers. The first was announced by Samuel Taylor Still (1828-1917) and the second by Daniel David Palmer (1845-1913). Though Chinese medical ideas had been introduced to Europe in the seventeenth century and then attracted sporadic interest in Continental countries, the western practice of acupuncture only became frequent some fifteen years after the establishment of the Peoples' Republic of China in 1949.

Chiropractors and osteopaths hold their begetters dear and the ancient texts (or glosses of them) are central to acupuncture education. In this chapter I outline the ideas of Still and Palmer, and some of the concepts associated with traditional acupuncture practice.

TURNING BACK

In a 1914 paper about new art movements, T.E. Hulme suggested that the first attempt to formulate a different attitude involved a return to archaism. The geometrical, abstract arts of the past were re-emerging and supplanting the soft and vital lines of organic forms which had held sway since the Renaissance. Absolutely distinct in kind, each sprang from and corresponded to a certain general attitude to the world and to the human relation to nature. The humanistic consciousness placed man at the centre of the world. By contrast, the tendency towards geometrical abstraction was necessary to express a certain intensity, creating a separation of the durable and permanent from the danger, flux and impermanence of outside nature:

> The need which art satisfies here, is not the delight in the forms of nature, which is characteristic of all vital arts, but the exact contrary. In the reproduction of natural objects there is an attempt to purify them of their characteristically living qualities in order to make them necessary and immovable. The changing is translated into something fixed and necessary. This leads to rigid lines and dead crystalline forms, for pure geometrical regularity gives a certain pleasure to men troubled by the obscurity of outside appearances (Hulme, 1960, 86).

A return to the archaic, Hulme said, was reinforced by the difficulty in finding immediately an appropriate method of expression. In the beginnings of a movement, the artist felt he must have done with the contemporary means but another and more fitting method was not easily created: 'The way from intention to expression does not come naturally, as it were from in outwards' (p. 99).

New systems of medicine — conveying different interpretations of the sources, meaning and treatment of bodily disorder — are similarly informed. While a radically different approach might be dismissed as regressive and opposed to contemporary understandings (which, in Hulme's sense, is accurate enough but no more than a denial), it signifies an alteration to the world attitude — from faith in the capability to master nature by inductive reasoning to the deductive certitudes of structural abstraction in the face of nature's confusions and dangers. The necessary medical presupposition, as Hulme had said of abstract arts, is the idea of disharmony or separation between humankind and the harshness of the outside world.

Histories of alternative medicines often start with accounts of the unhappy condition of orthodox practice at the time of their introduction (see Kaufman, 1971, for homeopathy in America, and Nicholls, 1988, for homeopathy in Britain; Wardwell, 1992, for chiropractic; and Gevitz, 1982, for osteopathy). The idea is that alternatives emerge in response to the apprehension of medical barbarism and ineptitude, and are successful to the degree that patients share the opinion that gentler methods are to be preferred to bloodletting, blistering, purging and the like. But the appearance of a new medicine is no mere reflex. Another view of the world is expressed. Suffering, the uncertainty of life and incapability in the face of its disorder yield an espousal of the regulated.

Consider A.T. Still's account of his turning-point. In 1864, two of his children and an adopted child died of spinal meningitis over a few days. Still says that when he gazed upon them:

> I propounded to myself the serious question, 'In sickness has not God left man in a world of guessing? Guess what is the matter? What to give and guess the result? And when dead, guess where he goes'. I decided then that God was not a guessing God, but a God of truth (Still, 1897, 99).

Still was fortified by a surety that the body was ordered in accordance with God's absolute law. He 'flung to the breeze the banner of Osteopathy' ten years later, on 22 June 1874, but in-between he pursued notions of mechanical exactitude. After inventing a reaper and a milk churn he began:

> an extended study of the drive-wheels, pinions, cups, arms, and shafts of human life, with their forces, supplies, framework, attachments by ligaments, muscles, their origin and insertion; − I believed that something abnormal could be found in some of the nerve divisions which would tolerate a temporary or permanent suspension of the blood either in arteries or veins, and cause disease (1908, 93-94).

Palmer also arrived at a certitude. He said that from the dim ages of the past, man had searched for an antidote, but to no avail. The question that had always been uppermost in his mind as he searched for the cause of disease, Palmer went on, was why one person became afflicted and another did not:

> **Why?** What difference was there in the two persons that caused one to have pneumonia, catarrh, typhoid or rheumatism, while his

partner, similarly situated, escaped? **Why?** This question had worried thousands for centuries and was answered in September 1895 (D.D. Palmer, 1910, 17-18).

Still found his answer when he switched, first, from orthodox practice to the laying on of hands in magnetic healing and then (in the 1870s) to the use of them to manipulate. Likewise, Palmer turned from nine years practice as a magnetic healer to spinal adjustment after the September 1895 discovery that settled his questioning — the relief of a case of deafness, and then one of heart trouble, by 'racking' vertebrae back into position:

> Then I began to reason if two diseases, so dissimilar as deafness and heart trouble, came from impingement, a pressure on nerves, were not other diseases due to similar cause? Thus the science (knowledge) and art (adjusting) of Chiropractic were formed at that time. I then began a systematic investigation for the cause of all diseases and have been amply rewarded (1910, 18-19).

The western adoption of traditional Chinese medicine (TCM as it is called) also was accompanied by a sense of re-discovery and innovation amongst those who took it up in a wholesale way. The espousal of an answer from the past and from elsewhere went hand-in-hand with the identification of unsatisfactory features of contemporary medical practice. Yet TCM was considered to be thoroughly modern. Advocates detected a link between Chinese mystical traditions and advanced science, especially contemporary physics, which had itself (so it was believed) turned into a transcendental exploration.

Therapeutic actions are prosaic and may be performed in an empirical fashion. Anybody might stick in needles but only traditional acupuncturists used a complex of embracing theory that invested signs with their meaning and enabled point selections to counter the disarrayed influences. The key to understanding lay in the works of the old masters, the sages who had plumbed the depths of bodily operations. Traditional Chinese medicine paid heed to its history, something, the adepts said, that practitioners of the allegedly scientific medicine of the West had ignored.

A return is justified, often after the event, by a turning away from what is. The extant scheme of things is said to have had its day, and the turning back is heralded as an innovation. Samuel Hahnemann (1755-1843), who resurrected the principle of similars in 1790 and enunciated homeopathy from 1810 onwards in successive editions of his *Organon of Medicine*, said that in earlier times there had sprung up:

> a mode of treatment with mixtures of unknown medicinal substances for forms of disease arbitrarily set up, and directed towards some material object completely at variance with nature and experience, hence, as may be supposed, with a bad result — such is old medicine, *allopathy* as it is termed (Hahnemann, 1988, 31).

Still and Palmer wrote similarly. Having established osteopathy, Still concluded that the medicine he had formerly practised was a bodily imposition made in the name of a false deity:

> Allopathy — builded its temples to the god who purged, puked, perspired, opiated, drank whiskey and other stimulants; destroyed in thousands, ruined nations, established whiskey saloons, opium dens, insane asylums, naked mothers and hungry babies, and still cries aloud, and says: 'Come unto me and I will give you rest. I have opium, morphine, and whiskey by the barrel' (Still, 1899, 208).

'Think of a Chiropractor substantially conquering disease!', Palmer wrote (1910, 71), 'that expression sounds Allopathic'. The system he had developed after giving the first chiropractic adjustment in September 1895 was:

> destined to revolutionize the Old School methods of practice which have been in vogue 2,000 years. There have been, and are today many methods of treating diseases, each and every one built on the old-time notion that disease is an evil, an entity which must be driven out, made to vacate, and the system cleansed of impurities before health can be restored; that cancers, body and skin diseases are efforts on the part of Nature to rout the enemy and that inflammation and fever are purifiers (D.D. Palmer, 1910, 74).

Hahnemann (1988, 31) maintained that previous medical systems were not consonant with nature and experience. They were 'mere theoretical webs, woven by cunning intellects out of pretended consequences'. Natural diseases were mistakenly located and arbitrarily classified by their organic causes. They had been established as things with opposing remedies but in nature no cure ever took place by the introduction of an alien morbid state. Diseases consisted 'solely of the sufferings of the patient, and the sensible alterations in his health, in a word, solely of the totality of the symptoms, by means of which the disease demands the medicine requisite for its relief'. They were 'purely dynamic deranging irritations of the vital force' which were to be overcome by introducing similar deranging irritations (1988, 157-159).

Palmer and Still also began their expositions with the question: what is disease? And each, like Hahnemann, turned disease on its head. Still held (1910, 21) that disease was simply an effect. So did Palmer:

> I am well aware that Chiropractic is a new departure, that adjusting causes is a radical change from treating effects, that it is making a greater inroad in the old methods than any other method; but I care not, so long as I know that I am right (D.D. Palmer, 1910, 100).

The old school looked upon disease as an interloper but now it was construed as an expression of the interior state, a swaying above or below normalcy. As Palmer had it (1910, 18-19), his discovery had unlocked the secrets of functional metabolism: diseases were 'conditions resulting from an excess or deficiency of functionating'.

Like Hahnemann, Still and Palmer did not offer alternatives but medicine itself, liberated from the nosological bondage that age had accreted. Each claimed their authority from Nature and their lineage from antiquity. The discontinuity lay with the allopaths who ignored or had forgotten their progenitors: allopathy had strayed, not homeopathy, chiropractic and osteopathy. The originators did not renounce science but claimed it. The body had been adjusted from time immemorial, Palmer noted, but he was the one who had made a science out of it; and science was 'knowledge reduced to law and embodied in a system' (1910: 741).

Even as these medicines ran with the grain of modernity, they conveyed different understandings of the human situation and of the connections between it and the powers in Nature. Chiropractic, osteopathy and traditional acupuncture were founded in metaphysical conceptions but their schemes were exact and applied. All three, like surgery, required dexterity. At the very time when medical technology had begun its ascendancy (see Reiser, 1978), Still and Palmer made hand-work into the source of healing.

Chiropractors, osteopaths and traditional acupuncturists stayed with old ways. The heartland operations, those deemed essential to each medicine and so constitutive of its distinct *practice*, made direct contact with the body. Unlike the penetrating handicraft of surgery, chiropractors and osteopaths applied variable pressure or directed surface force. Like surgical implements, the traditional acupuncturists' needles penetrated the skin. The intrusion might be slight by comparison but it was considered to be every bit as significant.

In sum, being sick and getting better were to be understood in other ways. Nature conferred healing prowess on those who restored bodily functions by aligning vital natural forces. 'We do not talk about the illnesses of people but patterns of disharmony', the acupuncture teacher told his class of beginners. From Palmer and Still onwards, chiropractors and osteopaths also have talked about health as harmony and disease — called 'dis-ease' by Palmer — as interrupting a natural order of geometrical regularity.

THE TENETS

Still knew he had got to the bottom of disease:

> The cause can be found and does exist in the limited or excited action of the nerves which control the fluids of part or the whole of the body. It appears perfectly reasonable to any person born above the condition of an idiot, who has familiarized himself with anatomy and its working with the machinery of life, that all diseases are mere effects, the cause being a partial or complete failure of the nerves to properly conduct the fluids of life (1908, 94).

Therefore osteopaths were obliged to maintain health rather than to cure disorder. As Still enjoined his followers:

> Your duty as a master mechanic is to know that the engine is kept in a perfect condition, so that there will be no functional disturbance to any nerve, or vein, or artery — Your osteopathic knowledge has surely taught you that, with an intimate acquaintance with the nerve- and blood- supply, you can arrive at a knowledge of the hidden cause of disease (1902, 70).

That put the operatives in command:

> A locomotive Engineer each Osteopath doth stand,
> And guides his engine, mortal man, with true un-erring hand;
> With master touch he doth adjust this engine's every part —
> Nerves, muscles, bones and ligaments and e'en the throbbing heart.

This science is exact and in accordance with its law
Each organ is revivified and acts without a flaw.

(From 'A letter to Mrs. Enquirer from Mrs. Experience', by
'Teddie'. In the second edition of A.T. Still's *Autobiography*, 1908,
294).

The medicine was to be drugless. In a speech on his sixty-ninth
birthday (1908: 340-346) Still said that since God's works were perfect
and trustworthy, He did not need any help 'and did not make man's
stomach to be a slop-pail for either dope or pills, big or little'. God
was no drug doctor: if He was competent and knew His business then
He certainly had made a good job of man. Still would try to work the
machine as God had formulated it. The discovery of osteopathy, so
he understood, had been put into his hand by the God of nature. 'I
am what some people call "inspired"', Still said, but 'we Methodists
call it "intuitive"'.

Still's conception of the body as an engine with God as its
artificer was not new. Boyle, Hobbes and others in the seventeenth
century, saw the Maker's hand made plain in the laws of matter and
local motion and in mechanic regularity.[1] Still also used a social
figure. The body was like a well-organised city:

> Each organ is a laborer of skill and belongs to the union of Perfect
> Work. Each laborer or organ must be in perfect health, or some
> degree of failure, a beginning of universal shortage in perfect work
> throughout the system or city will result — Just as a filthy sewer will
> produce disease in the whole city, so the failure of one organ will
> produce disease in the whole body, and the salvation of the city or
> body, depends on your mechanical philosophy and work (Still,
> 1910, 20).

The body as a whole was a functionary with duties to perform and
the organs were functionaries with duties to the body (1910, 21).
There was the social order of the body and the higher order of its
culminating state: 'If the body is the empire of the living man', Still
said, 'how large is the emperor? Is it necessary for him to be as large
as the whole empire?' (1910, 379). Was not the house much larger
than the lady who presided over and governed it? Still concluded: 'My
opinion is that organized life in man or beast is very small and is the
power behind the throne of man's physical body' (1910, 379).

Hobbes analogised in the reverse direction. Man, by his Art
(imitating God's Art in making nature), created the State 'which is

but an Artificiall Man' (1985, 81). In which case, the State was but an imperfect human extension of God's contrivance. But Still rather gave the impression that God stood behind the social order as He did behind the body. Still was no radical in politics: he had nothing to say about social conditions.

In close to a thousand pages of his 1910 *Textbook of the Science, Art and Philosophy of Chiropractic for Students and Practitioners*, also called *The Chiropractor's Adjuster*, Daniel David Palmer passed back and forth between expositions of his medicine, condemnations of his son Bartlett Joshua Palmer (1881-1961) and others for misappropriating chiropractic and corrections to their misrepresentations of it, poems, repetitions, extracts from newspapers and much else besides. This remarkable mixture was published four years after D.D. Palmer dissolved his interest in the college in Davenport, Iowa, that he had founded in 1897. B.J. Palmer, who graduated from it in 1902, edged his father out (Wardwell, 1992, 60) and remained in firm command for over fifty years.

The Chiropractor's *Adjuster* was not D.D. Palmer's first book. *The Science of Chiropractic* was jointly issued with his son in 1906 but D.D. Palmer said he had written nearly all the contents (1910, 913). The next edition, dated 1906-1910, carried B.J. Palmer's name alone. In a historical section (1906-1910, 11) he said that after his father gave the 'first accidental crude adjustment' in September 1895, the growth of chiropractic:

> remained practically dormant till 1903, since which time, his son B.J. Palmer, D.C., Ph.C.[Doctor of Chiropractic, Philosopher of Chiropractic], has developed it into a well defined non-therapeutical philosophy, science and art that has no resemblance whatever to any therapeutical method.

D.D. explained (1910, 605): 'because of an avaricious longing, the desire grew within him to possess the credit rightfully belonging to another, so that he might be IT'. And complained (p. 915): 'He has mutilated my writings and misrepresented the facts, laying himself liable to the United States courts for a $100 fine for each article appropriated by him'.

B.J. is even held responsible for his father's demise — his car having hit D.D. during a college homecoming parade on 20 August 1913. Having noted that D.D. left the day after the accident for

California and that his death there on 20 October 1913 is recorded as due to typhoid fever, Wardwell (1992, 62) comments:

> Whether B.J. contributed to his father's death as alleged, there is little doubt that, although he always paid formal tribute to his father as the 'discoverer of chiropractic', he could be considered as having 'symbolically killed' his father by taking PSC (the Palmer School of Chiropractic) away from him, removing D.D.'s name from the title page of later editions of their *Science of Chiropractic*, and taking full credit for himself as the 'developer of chiropractic' in directions that D.D. rejected.

Gibbons (1980b, 9-10) says that 'largely unsubstantiated charges of patricide would linger for years'. They did not so much linger as amplify the creation legend by building on D.D.'s own complaints about his son's emulation. According to this version, B.J. divided chiropractic and retarded its just recognition by distorting his father's healing message. Chiropractors of this persuasion still will say that B.J. killed his father. Also he is charged with getting rid of D.D.'s original work. A Phillip teacher commented (Terrett, 1986, 156):

> It was in the year 1910 that this book [*The Chiropractor's Adjuster*] was published, but all copies were quickly bought up and destroyed. You could not get a copy any place, at any price, after the first issue came out. In fact, you could not find a copy for 'love or money'. The leaders of the profession at that time did not want the world to know anything about the teachings of old Dr. Daniel D. Palmer. . . . With the effective suppression/disappearance of D.D. Palmer's book, the early leaders then greatly distorted their founder's science, philosophy and vision for chiropractic, as the book wasn't reprinted for half a century, some five years after B.J. Palmer's death.

While he said that he had formulated 'quite a portion of what now constitutes Chiropractic' during the previous nine years (that is, when he was practising as a magnetic healer), D.D. dated his discovery to September 1895 when he adjusted the back of a negro janitor and restored his hearing (1910, 18, 101).

The elder Palmer maintained that chiropractic was not a therapeutic system. Therapeutics was:

> that branch of medical science which considers the application of remedies as a means of cure. As Chiropractors do not use medicine

and have no need for remedies, therefore Chiropractic is not therapeutical; has no resemblance to any therapeutic system (D.D. Palmer, 1910, 143).

D.D. conceived a universe of spirit and matter, with life being 'but the expression of spirit thru matter' (1910, 495). It followed from his contrast of the vital life force and physical forces that he saw man as 'composed of intelligence and matter, spirit and material, the mortal and immortal, the everlasting and the transient. These two entities are linked together by the bond of union — the soul — intelligent life' (1910, 491).

The *outward* expression of that intelligence, which he called Educated, was made evident by the senses and manifested its functions in securing the means to physical survival. Then there was the Innate. This form of intelligence, which was also known (though inadequately, he believed) as 'Nature, intuition, instinct, spirit, and sub-conscious mind', maintained the *inner* physical order and was:

a segment of that Intelligence which fills the universe. This universal, All Wise, is metamerized, divided into metameres as needed by each individualized being. This somatome of the whole, never sleeps nor tires, recognizes neither darkness nor distance and is not subject to material laws or conditions. It continues to care for and direct the functions of the body as long as the soul holds body and spirit together (1910, 491-492).

Hence, Innate Intelligence gave expression to and was the guiding principle of universal order:

Innate — born with. And so far I would not change it except to replace it with the name of that individualized entity which really is a part or portion of that All Wise, Almighty, Universal Intelligence, the Great Spirit, the Greek's Theos, the Christian's God, the Hebrew's Helohim, the Mahometan's Allah, Hahnemann's Vital Force, new thot's [sic] Divine Spark, the Indian's Great Spirit, Hudson's Subconscious Mind, the Christian Scientist's All Goodness, the Allopath's Vis Medicatrix Naturae — the healing power of nature (1910, 493).

In contrast to the inductivism of Educated Intelligence, which started as a blank and died with the body, Innate Intelligence gave rise to a deductive vital science; for if the Innate had normal control of all bodily actions then 'the functions which perform all of these acts may be modified — increased or decreased — by the alterations of tissue' (1910, 495). Distortions of the inductive principle perturbed the inner (normal) work of Innate Intelligence: 'Thus, Innate would run functions physiologically, while Educated with a perverted mind would make them pathological' (1910, 497).

Palmer shifted easily from metaphysical categories to neurophysiological constructs. Motor and sensory impulses were transmitted by molecular vibration (1910, 188). These impulses were the medium of Innate transmission. Nerve impingements caused all the trouble. They resulted from minute vertebral displacements, called subluxations by D.D. in order to distinguish them from the luxations known to allopathic medicine (1910, 69). The correction or adjustment of subluxations allowed the innate to continue with its business. 'I founded the science and art of Chiropractic on the plan of economy, not elaboration' said Palmer. 'The act of replacing vertebrae, is that of racking into normal position those which have been displaced by traumatism or poisons' (1910, 69).

Here was a sure way of enabling the Innate to get on with its proper task:

The Chiropractor teaches that all organs must agree,
That all must work together in most perfect harmony.
Thus, when all regulate the spine its functions to fulfill,
All other parts experiences alike responsive thrill.

The kidneys, lungs and liver and the spleen and heart and brain
Are organs linked together by the sympathetic chain
And from a common center, they one and all obtain
A regulative, guiding free that makes their duty plain.

Adjustment, regulation is all that we require.
It lifts the baneful pressure that smothers vital fire,
Gives freedom to the muscles that they may freely act,
And the body perfect liberty to functionate intact.

Away with drugs which poison and instruments that kill.
Let us use, in wisdom's way, of mental, manual skill.
The hands, by mind directed, can drive our ills away
And bring us advantageous health for which we all shall pray

(From 'Chiropractic', by W.J. Colville, in D.D. Palmer, 1910, 22)

Like Still, Palmer emphasised the principle of functional order, with disease resulting from the excessive or insufficient performance of functions (1910, 140). He said that while some applied disease to structural change and disorder to functional derangement, 'It is a self-evident fact that normal structure and normal functions are co-existent' (1910: 569). Nevertheless, he was more inclined to functional interpretations. When impingements were removed, the vital energy of the body performed functions at will.[2]

Palmer went to great lengths to distinguish chiropractic from osteopathy. Since he came to hold that the body was informed by an active power — being operated by the individualisation of universal spirit in intelligent life — he took strong exception to Still's assertion that man was a machine. Palmer saw no resemblance or likeness between a machine and the human body: 'A machine is an unimpassioned, automatic contrivance, composed of mechanical elements. The body is a self conscious, appreciative, animated being' (1910, 128). He exclaimed:

> The body a machine! Altered blood flow causes the machine to be erratic in its movements! Such is Osteopathy and I am sorry to know that many, very many Chiropractors have absorbed so much of Osteopathy which they try to palm off as Chiropractic (1910, 141).

Palmer also criticised osteopathy because its adherents used 'orthopaedical machines, drugs and surgery' (1910, 465). The principles of osteopathy and allopathy were the same and their practices differed only in degree: the allopaths were more medical and less mechanical while the osteopaths were more mechanical and less medical (1910: 609). Besides, osteopaths were inclined to regard disease as natural, that is, as an expression of the body's own curative process. There was one osteopath (unnamed but certainly not Still) who said that 'Smallpox is renovating, while vaccination is contaminating', eliciting from Palmer: 'Don't that jar your mother's preserves? Smallpox a zymotic, filth [sic] disease renovating? No person is improved by being poisoned by either smallpox or vaccination' (1910, 717).

The way Palmer saw it is neatly summed up in 'Don't Blame it on the Devil', an unattributed poem in his book. A verse reads:

> It is known that sin is but disease, a weakness of the mind,
> All ailments, indisposition and sickness one can find,
> Are but results of vertebral displacements which unhinge
> The nerves which chiropractors by adjustments find impinged

> (1910, 130).

Palmer held that diseases could be traced to a sole origin. He said —
it is the single item extracted from his writings that is most quoted by
critics to damn chiropractic as a whole — that 95 per cent of diseases
were caused by displaced vertebrae. He held that luxated joints other
than the backbone caused the other 5 per cent (1910, 100).

Palmer's conviction may be compared with that of the dean of
the Phillip school of chiropractic and osteopathy:

> We at Phillip (and the vast majority of chiropractors) do not
> embrace a dogma that 'the treatment of the spine (can cure)
> systemic diseases'.

> In addition to disorders which may be identified as clearly musculo-
> skeletal (e.g. back injury), we do know we have success in the
> treatment of a group of pathophysiological disorders of a functional
> nature, including certain types of asthma, persistent headaches and
> migraine.

> We also successfully treat many patients who come to us after
> having been misdiagnosed by others as suffering from a variety of
> systemic disorders, creating an impression that a musculo-skeletal
> disorder was actually something else.

> But, as chiropractors, we treat on the basis of our own diagnosis —
> and we diagnose and treat primarily musculo-skeletal disorders.[3]

The dean was responding to a physiotherapy educator who was
quoted as repudiating any association between her occupation and
one whose dogma was that treatment of the spine could cure systemic
disease. Not that physiotherapists ignored the significance of the
Innate. One wrote in a physiotherapy journal editorial: 'It would
appear that all physiotherapists, irrespective of their level of
experience, have an innate sense of what constitutes quality and can
recognise it' (Bromley, 1987, 153).

Traditional Chinese medicine (TCM) has no simple and
unilinear history. It was influenced by and gave expression to
conflicting schools of philosophical and scientific thought. (See Lu
Gwei-Djen and Needham 1980 for a history of acupuncture; Schwartz
1985, for ancient Chinese philosophies; and Unschuld 1985, for a
history of Chinese medical ideas.) There is about as much sense in
referring to TCM as an entity as there is in talking similarly about
European science and philosophy. But historical, cultural and
geographic particularities are set aside in order to divide the world
into East and West.

Even so, in the received form in which it is now applied outside China and surrounding countries by those who call themselves traditional acupuncturists or practitioners of traditional Chinese medicine, there are common understandings of the sources, manifestations, and progress of bodily conditions. The medicine has its language, not complete and suffering in translation but sufficiently distinct to identify those who use it.

The reading of diagnostic signs (especially in the pulses and the tongue) and the interpretation of their meaning demand subtlety and alertness. The purpose of treatment, by whatever means, is to maintain or restore a unique balance that is intimately connected to the cosmos. The principal of the Melbourne college said of traditional Chinese medicine 'It's a functional medicine that tries to re-establish a harmonious function of the whole. It's pre-pathology, preventive. The pathology is the result of untreated organic disease'.

Acupuncture is one method of achieving this end. Needles are implanted, singly or more often in combination, at defined surface points, to specified depths, for certain periods and at designated times of the day, season or year. For the same purpose, but perhaps more usually for use in chronic conditions, a tinder made from the leaves of an East Asian wormwood, *Artemisia moxa*, is burnt on or near defined surface points which usually coincide with acupuncture points, for defined periods and frequencies and at defined intensities.

Kleinman (1986, 193) said that 'Most non-Western societies conceive the body as mindful, the mind as embodied'. Chinese medicine, the version of it taught in the acupuncture colleges, depended on contrasting a western style of medical thinking about the corporeal human substance with a conception which drew much of its inspiration from Taoist thought. As the students in the acupuncture college were often reminded, they had to escape from their usual western understanding of the body and to learn to think about it in another way.

Was there a single other way? Unschuld (1985, 57) suggested that one of the characteristic traits of the history of ideas in Chinese medicine was the continuous tendency, but within limits, toward a syncretism with practitioners and thinkers liberally applying all the concepts available:

Whenever antagonistic subparadigms emerged within one of the major paradigms, the resulting contradictions appear to have been solved only rarely, if ever, in a manner familiar to the historian of medicine and science in the West . . . after a while the issue was resolved neither in a dialectical sense in that a more advanced synthesis was created out of thesis and antithesis nor in a (Kuhnian) revolutionary sense in that a more recent paradigm achieved prevalence and dominated a subsequent era of 'normal science' until it was replaced by the next revolutionary paradigm.

That was a difficult idea to get across to students. They expected consistency and an organised structure. It was not so much that the ideas were alien but that they did not fit together as they should. One way in which the organs were brought into a coherence is to be found in the most famous of Chinese medical books, the *Nei Jing* (or Yellow Emperor's Book of Internal Medicine), a compendium of texts of Confucian, Taoist and earlier origin (dated between the second century B.C. and the eighth century A.D). The *Su Wen* ('Simple Questions') section has the mythical Emperor *Huang Di* asking the physician *Ch'i Bo* the functions of the five organs, the six bowels and the twelve vessels (or meridians as they are now frequently called). The reply starts:

> The Heart is a royal organ; it represents the King; in it resides the Spirit.
> The Lungs are the ministers; they rule the energy of the exterior, of the skin.
> The Liver is the general who works out the plans.
> The Gall Bladder is the judge who decides and condemns.
> The Envelope of the Heart represents the civil servants; from them can come joy and pleasure.

(Chinese Medical Classics 1979, 24)

Unschuld suggested (1987, 1027) that an image of society and national economy was transferred to a perception of the structure and workings of the interior of the body. He noted elsewhere (1985, 67) that in its beginnings, the principles that dominated the system of healing 'corresponded closely to the social-political order advocated during the same period by Confucian political ideology'. Durkheim and Mauss (1969) argued that Chinese thought was a projection of the extant categories of social organisation. But the connection ran in both directions. The idea of correspondences influenced thinking about the State: Confucian political doctrine incorporated theories, on which the medicine was also based, to explain the rise and decline of the dynasties (Unschuld, 1985, 65). Nevertheless, the due place of and the fitting relation between the organs of the state could be established in terms of bodily organs and their functional exchanges. The social order explained the body, as in the *Nei Jing*, and the body was used to legitimate the social order.

Any attempt at a synopsis of the vast body of Chinese philosophical and scientific knowledge would be facile. The many volumes of Needham's *Science and Civilization in China* (1954-1988) are indispensable for this purpose. Two items will be mentioned to inform the subsequent account: the concept of *ch'i* (in the Wade-Giles romanisation) or Qi (in more recent use) and that of Yin-Yang. Their relevance here lies in a belief in the congruence of modern western and ancient Chinese concepts. Also, teachers had the problem of conveying an understanding of them in familiar English terms. In ordinary college shorthand use, Qi meant energy which flowed through the meridians (that is, the passages of its activity) and Yin-Yang referred to the vital balance of energies (not, it should be emphasised, to a simple dichotomy).

Unschuld (1985, 71-72) traced the origins of Qi to the pictogram indicating 'vapors rising from rice (or millet: i.e. from food)'. Qi referred to influences within and without the body. It came very early to designate dispersible vapors floating through the air and, together with blood, through the organism. Therefore Unschuld translated Qi as '"finest matter influence" or simply "influence", with a substance or matter connotation in mind'. Needham (1962 vol. 2, 472) preferred to leave Qi untranslated since its significance for Chinese authors (nearly everyone who addressed Nature used it) could not be conveyed by a single English word. He went on to say of Qi: 'It could be a gas or vapour, but also an influence as subtle as those which "aetherial waves" or "radioactive emanations" have implied for modern minds'.

The significance of all this lies in the common representation of Qi as an immaterial principle or mystical abstraction because no evidence can be found to demonstrate its empirical existence. The issue, in short, concerns the 'reality' of Qi and of its supposed meridian routes. While reports on acupuncture by Australia's National Health and Medical Research Council did not single out Qi or any other theoretical aspect for attention, traditional knowledge was dismissed on this ground:

> In the face of research developments there is no need for romantic or fanciful explanations of the basis of acupuncture analgesia. It is not necessary to invoke models involving meridians or other mystical explanations (Westerman 1988, 1989, 14).

While such a criticism might be countered by arguing the materiality of Qi, this also misses the point. The dispute is not over translation but over a variety of conceptual applications in a transported cultural scheme. The use of the western concept of energy to interpret the Chinese concept of Qi, Unschuld argued (1987, 1024), 'mirrors a western quest for an alternative [to western understandings] that remains, nevertheless, within the limits of basic western values'.

The theory of Yin-Yang emerged from the ancient idea of systematic likenesses or correspondences, what Frazer (1911, 52) called homeopathic or imitative magic. This might be taken to consign Yin-Yang, like Hahnemann's principle of similars, to false science. But the whole idea is to convey an encompassing reciprocity. As the acupuncture college students were told, the signs for Yin and Yang meant the shady side of the hill and the sunny side of the hill; that is, they indicated the differences of cold-heat, drawing in-bursting out, interior-exterior, female-male, lower-upper, earth-heaven, and so on. Certain organs were designated as Yin organs and others as Yang, just as external influences were one or the other.

Yet there was an integration within this seeming duality. One was contained in the other: Yin was never entirely Yin nor Yang entirely Yang. Nor were the organs to be identified with those bearing the western names. They both were them and more than them. This may sound like a shadow-play with words but the intent was to capture a rhythmical ordering of the universe. In modern terms, Yin-Yang was said by traditional acupuncturists to be exemplified in the principles of biological periodicity (for example, the circadian order), in homeostasis and holism. Chiropractors and osteopaths also could identify their medicines with these principles. 'Homeostasis', a chiropractic teacher said, 'is our modern term for Innate Intelligence'.

Hence, supporters might believe that the concepts were part of the stock-in-trade of advanced science but continued to be distinctive of their medicine. The principal of the Melbourne college explained the uniqueness of traditional Chinese medicine by a contrast:

> In Chinese medicine the differentia are quite unlike western medicine. Integral to a diagnostic term in TCM is the cause: the term that describes a disease is a description of the cause. In western medicine you might say this patient has a migraine but I would say the person has liver Qi stagnating leading to Yang rising

— that is the actual path not just the name of the disease — it means a blockage of the body's energy within the liver channel.

Dispute abounded over the science of acupuncture. Some commentators said that in essence it was a mediaeval science (e.g. Lu Gwei-Djen and Needham, 1980, (xx), and 185, referring to the views of the French physician and acupuncturist, Khoubesserian). One of its leading established medical advocates maintained that Chinese medicine fulfilled all the criteria by which a true science could be distinguished (Porkert, 1988, 29). More than that, others asserted that acupuncture was as advanced as a science could be, due to the affinity of Taoism and modern physical theory. In a book recommended for reading by first year acupuncture college students (*The Tao of Physics*, Capra, 1976) it was suggested that:

> In Chinese philosophy, the field idea [i.e., quantum field theory] is not only implicit in the notion of the *Tao* as being empty and formless, and yet producing all forms, but is also expressed explicitly in the concept of *ch'i* . . . In the human body, the 'pathways of *ch'i*' are the basis of traditional Chinese medicine (1976, 236).

A traditional acupuncturist wrote in the local journal:

> It is interesting that Quantum Mechanics has come to the conclusion that, at the atomic level, 'Matter behaves both as particles and waves'. If acupuncture alters the waves circulating in the body, it is then possible that these changes could manifest in an alteration at the atomic or molecular level causing the physiological effect observed (Albon 1988, 20).

Kaptchuk, whose book *The Web That Has No Weaver* (1983) was another first year college text, thought likewise. Supporting the view that western medicine had yet to incorporate the achievements of the quantum revolution, he said: 'Even in the inner sanctum of health care, calls are being made for changes to new paradigms' (1983, 263).

CONCLUSION

Chiropractic, osteopathy and traditional acupuncture (in its recent western adoption) were founded around redemptive possibilities. The world of healing was in a mess. Medicine had mistaken the way but it could be transformed through the adoption of solutions that were at once novel and antique.

Sustaining appreciations of distinctiveness and purpose were tempered in the fires of condemnation and attempted suppression. But reactionary enmity was to be expected. Such was the character of the orthodox: they admitted of no exceptions. Which only showed that the worth of a medicine was confirmed by the persecution of its bearers. As Paracelsus said of his opponents (1990, 73-74):

> You are serpents and I expect poison from you. With what scorn have you proclaimed that I am the Luther of physicians, with the interpretation that I am a heretic — Who are Luther's foes? The very rabble that hates me. And what you wish him you wish me — to the fire with us both.

A band must form around evangels if their works are to endure. So it was with Still, Palmer, and the unnumbered Chinese sages who, incongruously, were made into paladins of a European medical transformation. One had to organise, fight *and* negotiate in order to keep a medicine going toward its due recognition. But teachings and practices were likely to be modified, even to be distorted, during the pursuit. Alterations to the original messages, and the institution of local branches of the three medicines, are the subject of the next chapter.

Notes

1. 'For what is the Heart, but a Spring; and the Nerves, but so many Strings; and the Joynts, but so many Wheeles, giving motion to the whole Body, such as was intended by the Artificer?', Hobbes, *Leviathan* (1985, 81). In likening the world to a rare clock, Boyle (1966, 152) combined his non-conformist religious belief and science in the same way as Still was to do. At the end of the eighteenth century William Godwin, for a short time a Presbyterian minister, maintained that the human mind was also a system of mechanism: 'understanding by mechanism nothing more than a regular succession of phenomena, without any uncertainty of event, so that every consequent requires a specific antecedent, and could be no otherwise in any respect than as the antecedent determined it to be' (Godwin, 1976, 360-361). He went on to conceive the body as 'so constituted as to be susceptible to vibrations, in the same manner as the strings of a musical instrument' — a figure that D.D. Palmer also used in his theory of tonicity which he held to be the basic principle of the science and philosophy of chiropractic (1910: 58, 659). However, Godwin maintained that thought — 'the medium through which the motions of the animal system are usually carried on' — was a mechanistic system of a different kind: 'The most powerful impression, either from without or within, constantly gets the better of its competitors, and forcibly drives out the preceding thought, till it is in the same irresistible manner driven out by its successor' (1976: 363, 376).

2. Concurrently, the structure-function relationship was being disputed in established medicine. Reiser (1981, 138-139) summarises the positions: 'Anatomical diagnosis, whether directed at lesions in the solid parts or fluids of the body, sought a locus for disease. It asked, "Where is the lesion?" Functional diagnosis sought to evaluate performance. It asked, "What can the organ do?" Those physicians who emphasized function disavowed the maxim of practice: when you find a lesion, treat it. The functionalist ministered only to defects that clearly threatened or interfered with the patient's activities'. Palmer and Still both regarded health as the performance of normal functions and they held similar views about the dysfunctional significance of lesions: Palmer (1910, 980) considered them to be the cause of functional derangements and Still (1910, 21-23) saw osteopathic lesions as the causes of friction which impeded the performance of the functionary duties of the brain, heart, venous and nervous systems.
3. Kleynhans, A. Letter to the Editor, 'Chiropractic is not a bar to amalgamation', *The Australian*, 19 September 1989.

III

THE PROGRESS OF MOVEMENTS

I really think that if everyone thought chiropractic was O.K., it would be just another way to get well. A lot of us through the years have suffered because of the law and a bad name and things like that, but that's the reason why a lot of us keep working so hard to bring people the truth

(American chiropractor, quoted in Cowie and Roebuck, 1975, 111).

EARLY DAYS

Still did not take long to introduce usual elements of medical education to the course he started in 1892. Surgery and obstetrics, as well as physiology, were added to anatomy and manipulation in 1896. Though marked by dispute, education and the scope of osteopathic practice were extended, culminating in the 1915 removal of a proscription against the teaching of *materia medica* (see Gevitz, 1982; 1988, for excellent accounts). American osteopathy inclined more and more toward regular practice over the next 60 years. Gevitz (1982, 141) cites a 1974 survey indicating that osteopaths used manipulation in less than 17 per cent of patient cases.

A few of Still's graduates were working in Melbourne in 1909. (For an abbreviated Australian history, see Hawkins and O'Neill, 1990.) No more than ten American-trained osteopaths, including a handful of Australians, were in practice at any one time in the years up to Second World War. They were isolated, condemned as quacks by the orthodox, and in danger of prosecution if they called themselves doctors. The absence of registration left them without the broad practice rights enjoyed by American osteopaths.

Though osteopathy was not registered in the United Kingdom, the British School of Osteopathy (BSO), founded in 1917, enjoyed considerable establishment (but not orthodox medical) esteem. This school and the more recent European School of Osteopathy, also in the United Kingdom, have stayed with Still's original no-drugs and all-manipulation platform. Perhaps British osteopaths did not aspire to assimilation or could not be tempted because the regular domain was so effectively closed against them (see Baer, 1984; 1987, about the separate development and professionalisation of British osteopathy).

Some Australian and overseas graduates of the British School of Osteopathy began to enter practice after the Second World War. Their occupational body, the Australian Osteopathic Association (AOA) which started in 1955, was tiny: it had 7 members when registration was first proposed in Victoria (Ward, 1975, 9) and 14 when the federal committee supported it in all the States (Webb, 1977, 41). Despite chiropractic endeavours to cut osteopathy out of the projected Victorian Act, the AOA lobbied hard and obtained a separate designation for osteopaths on the single register. This edged forward the case for an osteopathic degree, since the Webb committee linked registration to the provision of suitable local education. So small a group was most unlikely to get very far but the director of the Preston (later Phillip) Institute saw an opening and started to discuss possibilities with the AOA. In effect, the AOA, which had a member on the committee that was to decide chiropractic course location, also secured one for osteopathy by backing Preston's cause.[1] Though chiropractors and osteopaths played out the enmities to which their overseas training made them heir, they achieved their several purposes by backing each other. When the osteopathy course began six years later, it followed the BSO approach and employed its graduates.

Osteopathy entered Australia by another route. From the 1920s onwards, it was promoted as one amongst a number of therapies deemed safe and natural. Many private colleges offered osteopathy training alongside exercise, herbalism, nutritional practices and massage. Chiropractic and osteopathy were also taught together. Students could obtain certification in both and, not infrequently, in naturopathy as well. A shake-out occurred in the 1970s, brought on by the likelihood of chiropractic registration and resulting in the conversion of colleges and practitioners to chiropractic-only titles. Practitioner bonds remained as fragile as the colleges and occupational associations were numerous. The locals were held to be doctrinally promiscuous and educationally insufficient by the overseas-trained. Those who stuck by osteopathy, mainly in New South Wales, ended up with their own association, the United Osteopathic Physicians Guild (UOPG).

There is a large measure of UOPG support for the Phillip osteopathy programme. Nevertheless, the AOA and the UOPG remained apart during this study. Some AOA practitioners expressed concern about 'standards' and about being swamped in an amalgamation with the UOPG. They had much greater worries about being taken over by chiropractic. But a deal is a deal. Osteopathic continuity in Australia had been purchased at the expense of an association with chiropractic: the truce held, even as the sides to it kept up their convictions of superiority.

Gibbons (1980b, 12) says that B.J. Palmer controlled his chiropractic school to a suffocating degree. He 'jealously watched over the ideological flame, which he maintained he was to keep, and his financial judgment and decision making were absolute'. But B.J. 'would ultimately give chiropractic purpose, direction, and a distinct identity around which to gather and survive'.

B.J. translated his father's ideas into doctrine. He laid out (and initialled) 'The Master Key' of chiropractic in the following diagram:

Figure 1   Relationships between Innate and Educated

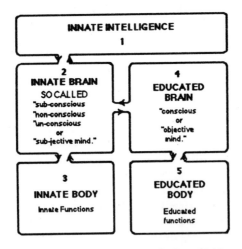

'The most valuable drawing in the world –

For it solves all the problems of man"

(B.J. Palmer, 1979, 55).

A chiropractor (Donahue 1986, 35) wrote about the difficulty with D.D. Palmer's teachings (which B.J.'s approach only magnified):

> The whole concept of innate of course rests on accepting on faith the basic premises without hope of any concrete proof. From a strictly scientific viewpoint, innate must be rejected out of hand because it fails the most fundamental requirement of science, namely testability. From the standpoint of logic, the whole concept of innate depends on the logical fallacy called word magic. Giving names and definitions to unprovable spiritual entities like innate and soul cannot guarantee their existence.

One of the fourth year Phillip chiropractic students thought likewise: 'I wonder whether [Innate and Universal Intelligence] are not the same as St. Thomas Aquinas was saying in the 12th century. Maybe it's just bad theology'.

The original fracture between father and son was compounded by many other disputes. Additional schools sprang up and disappeared as frequently in chiropractic as they did in osteopathy. B.J. Palmer, a tutiorist whose deductivism made the chiropractic principle into an immutable rule, was pitted against his latitudinarian opponents. He accused them of selling out on the Big Idea by mixing chiropractic with other methods of treatment. They denounced him for promoting schism by holding fast to rigid definitions of permissible action (B.J. called it pure and unadulterated or 'straight' chiropractic). More likely, his hardy band of followers required formulaic certainties of him and he was led to provide them by adopting the mantle of expositor. D.D. Palmer moved on so quickly that he did not become the slave of his disciples.[2]

Unlike osteopathy, where divisions turned on the assumption of orthodox medical practices, the chiropractic 'mixers' remained firmly opposed to drugs and surgery. Hence chiropractors, though they were riven by enduring contention, still represented chiropractic as radically pure overall. If they agreed about anything it was that their medicine had not attempted to gain acceptance by taking the compromising path of osteopathy.

American-trained chiropractors began to practise in Australia from around 1918 (see Campbell 1983, and Willis, 1983 for accounts). A national occupational body, the Australian Chiropractors' Association (ACA), was established in 1938. The fourteen subscribers belonged to B.J Palmer. At their preliminary meeting to consider establishing an association, Fraser, who became and remained president for twenty-four years 'stressed that the Association was for all 'straight' Chiropractors and would not cater for just one section of thought and hoped that all petty squabbles would be kept out'.[3]

Their constitution and rules provided that:

> no applicant shall be admitted as a member of the association who does not practise what is known to the profession as 'straight' Chiropractic and whose methods of dealing with patients for curative purposes are not strictly confined to the adjustment of the spine by the application of the bare hands without the addition of electro therapy, therapeutic lamps, use of instruments for curative purposes or any other method whatsoever, provided that this clause shall have no application to the recognised and well established practise of taking x-ray photos for the purposes of analysis (in Bolton, 1959, 8-9).

The new association kept its distance from the improprieties of local education. In 1940 a member pointed out that 'a certain Australian organisation was turning out so-called Chiropractors by a correspondence course'. The ACA decided to say nothing 'as this sort of thing would defeat itself'.[4] Restrictions were kept up. A member resigned in 1941, offering as reason 'the fact that he had undertaken other methods of practice which would conflict with our rules of Association'.[5] A membership candidate who had been practising as an osteopath and chiropractor was rejected but told that a further application would be considered at the end of the year 'provided he had put his house in order and during that time had practised "straight chiropractic"'.[6]

By the late 1960s, North American colleges were increasingly of the 'mixer' persuasion and their graduates were entering Australian practice and occupational politics. But 'straight' thinking did not fall away. The ACA did not so much change its doctrinal stripes as shift from an exclusive to an inclusive body as the membership qualification moved from adherence to an authorised chiropractic version to graduation from an authorised college: those in the U.S., the one in Canada and (later) the Anglo-European College in the U.K. Thereafter, hostilities were not ended but contained to the inner councils of the ACA.

The rival United Chiropractors Association of Australasia (UCA) was founded in 1961 to represent Victorian graduates of one of the local colleges but extended its cover to other Australian-trained practitioners through various amalgamations. Some in this camp 'saw themselves as osteopaths, naturopaths or acupuncturists, as much as chiropractors' (Campbell, 1983, 209). However, most had tied themselves firmly to chiropractic (even if they continued to 'mix' in their own way) by 1975 when the Ward Committee was investigating Victorian registration. The UCA supported colleges in Sydney and Melbourne and in 1975 the ACA started the International College of Chiropractic (ICC), forerunner of the Phillip school. The antagonism between the two associations was extreme, long-running and resolved along incorporative lines by their amalgamation in 1990 to form the Chiropractors' Association of Australia (National) (CAA(N)).

An earlier transfer of Victorian UCA members to the ACA says much about the modulation of principled differences in light of strategic imperatives. Earlier attempts to bring the associations together had failed, but in 1977, the Webb committee was about to recommend that the Australian states should register manipulative therapists and that an officially supported qualifying course of tertiary instruction in chiropractic should be established, probably in a Victorian college of advanced education. Victorian legislation to register chiropractors was ready to proceed and there was a sense of uncertainty and urgency. The ACA and UCA were fierce competitors for the course – education was of pivotal concern, both as an extension of occupational control and as a means to it.

Advanced education colleges also competed for chiropractic. The ACA backed the then Preston Institute of Technology which already had taken in the International College of Chiropractic (ICC) on a contract basis. The UCA and its affiliate, the Chiropractic College of Australia (CCA), supported the Royal Melbourne Institute of Technology (RMIT) and, when it pulled out of the race, the Lincoln Institute of Health Sciences. At the time, this college had a virtual state monopoly on the conduct of therapy (including physiotherapy) programmes.

The group that got the course and seats on the registration board was expected to cut out the opposition. The UCA had grounds for worry on this score: in Western Australia, the only state to have full chiropractic legislation at that time, ACA members controlled the licensing board and UCA members were unable to obtain registration (on the ground that their education was inadequate). Something similar might happen with training. Professional associations might not own higher education courses but no chiropractor had any illusions about the winner being able to influence appointments: the UCA would prefer its own sort and the ACA would stack the faculty with graduates from 'acceptable' overseas colleges.

The very strength of the animosity led ACA and UCA leaders to a negotiation: their calculations were informed by the fear each side had of losing to the other. The association between the CCA and RMIT 'put the wind up the ACA' according to one who was then a CCA student. Ironically, the UCA was worried about the precariousness of its RMIT connection.

In May 1977, just after the Webb report had been delivered but before its contents were made public, the head of the CCA (Fawke) had discussions with some naturopaths to discuss registration legislation. According to notes of the meeting, his assessment was that 'RMIT doesn't really want the [CCA] course because it is already overloaded. However RMIT doesn't want to lose by default'.[7] UCA leaders put out feelers for a discussion with the ACA.

When the two sides met, the major problems for chiropractic were identified as: (i) attacks by the Australian Medical and Physiotherapy Associations; (ii) obtaining chiropractic education at a tertiary level; and (iii) preparing the membership for registration and what followed from it.[8] The ACA representatives said their concerns were to get approval for a course at PIT and to maintain standards, both for entry to the profession and for the future. Those from the UCA said they wanted to secure practice privileges on a proper basis for their members (that is, they were concerned to avoid a repeat of the West Australian exclusion).

What emerged at the meeting was the renewed possibility of offering ACA membership to Victorian UCA members, an amalgamation with 'each side accepting the other's dead wood'. In summary, the conditions were that:

(i) [on the ACA side] the UCA members gave up the RMIT course proposal and supported the ICC/PIT proposal; they accepted provisional ACA membership to begin with and agreed to met assessment criteria after seminar attendance for full membership; and

(ii) [on the UCA side] there would be equal ACA/UCA membership on the registration board, UCA involvement in the ICC/PIT course, and participation on the ACA branch executive.

With these details spelt out, the pact was sealed. Fawke wrote to Lincoln and RMIT withdrawing UCA support for their course proposals, and to PIT offering unqualified support for its chiropractic programme.[9] PIT immediately wrote to the Victoria Institute of Colleges (VIC, the state co-ordinating body that would settle course location) conveying the 'pertinent information' that the amalgamated UCA/ACA had 'unreservedly given their support to the Chiropractic Programme being developed at the Preston Institute of Technology'. The acting director of PIT said helpfully that this would make the VIC decision on course siting 'much simpler'.[10]

The conflict between the ACA and the UCA had been as bitter as anything between chiropractic and medicine, and, indeed, federal leaders continued to pursue each other with great venom. But the justification for Victorian chiropractors coming together — the one given to Victorian ACA and UCA members — was the need for a united front in the face of the medical enemy. When Martin, the ACA's Victorian branch president, conveyed the merger resolution to members, he said:

> The ICC stands ready to help and it is now in my humble opinion, time for all chiropractors to stand up for unity. What keeps us apart is made up of both substance and illusion. Ten years from now and twenty years from now it will be a great vigorous independent profession if we stand together today and realise that what unites us far outweighs what divides us. The real enemy is manipulative therapy and the old guard of political medicine that almost reflexly opposes chiropractic. They can be a formidable force if we are not united in defence and in offence [sic]-FOR CHIROPRACTIC.[11]

Nobody wanted to be left out and the success of the Victorian ACA/UCA unity scheme lay in the insurance it provided to each side. The consensus between them, the thing they could agree about, was the antagonism of orthodox medicine but the ground on which they made alliance was their fear of each other.

Ten years later, as he surveyed the continuing warfare between chiropractors, both in America and in Australia, Martin remained convinced about the unity imperative and the reasons for it — 'If we don't get and stay united as a profession we deserve to be destroyed' — but he was less sure about the educational choice the ACA had made earlier when it was consulted about the development of the Lincoln course:

In Vic. in the mid seventies Graham Hunt and I were offered respectability and an enhanced new degree in Physiological Therapeutics and Specific Manipulative Therapy (this was pre PIT and pre-registration). In other words the same deal as this new DPT [Doctor of Physical Therapy] degree in the USA plus a large chiropractic content. As a variation of the Cyriax plan we turned it down in the name of D C's [Doctors of Chiropractic] everywhere.

Were we right? Do we deserve to continue as an independent profession? Sometimes as I read our journals and listen to my colleagues — I wonder . . . Who will offer a Chiropractic alternative after we destroy ourselves?[12]

People in movements are imbued with a determination to ensure the survival as well as the advancement of their ideas and practices. The principal of the Sydney acupuncture college explained why she and her Melbourne colleague were endeavouring to have their courses transferred to universities:

We are not doing it for ego or for a job for money. You have to have belief in your own cause. We are giving it to them because if it goes into a system there is a certain inertia, a status quo. That will protect it. If we die there may be others who will sell it out. We are just worried that it be preserved.

What had to be protected was the uncontaminated medical essence. Traditional acupuncturists knew their enemy: not only did established medicine assert monopoly rights to the subject but also it debased the central teachings by reducing acupuncture merely to an empirical practice. Then again, acupuncture had to be protected from the many other pretenders to knowledge of it — like chiropractors and naturopaths — and from those who let the side down most by purporting to represent it. Traditional acupuncturists could be their own worst enemies.

Opponents of registration and the higher education of traditional acupuncturists — such as the Australian Medical Acupuncture Society (AMAS), an association of some registered medical practitioners using acupuncture — distinguished 'non-medical' or 'lay' acupuncturists as the object of their condemnation. They contrasted the protection afforded by the scientific knowledge and education of 'proper' doctors with the dangers of getting acupuncture from anyone else.[13] Similarly, traditional acupuncturists could use the insufficient-training argument to lump competitors in other occupations together.

Distinguishing true bearers of the traditional acupuncture flame was another matter. For this purpose, considerations of doctrinal purity were increasingly supplanted by the adoption of the features that were likely to settle occupational registration. As with chiropractic and osteopathy years before, traditional acupuncture groups competed against each other for the privilege. Therefore it was important for representatives to demonstrate that their group was to be preferred because it was nationally representative, required practitioners to have a solid grounding in western science education, kept up ethics, had an associated but independent body that appraised course standards.

All the many Australian colleges and associations with a finger in the traditional acupuncture pie were preoccupied about the maintenance of principled distinctiveness and about surviving. They adjusted their affiliations and training accordingly. How far to modify without compromising? What was essential? Traditional acupuncture changed as traditional acupuncturists advanced. A message is constantly re-interpreted and a movement is never still.

WHAT MAKES ALTERNATIVES ALTERNATIVE?

Around the time when chiropractic registration was being sought, most Australian practitioners would have held that their occupation did offer a systematic alternative to much of (and some would have said to all of) standard medical practice. At the very least, chiropractors were near-united in believing that their care offered an alternative to much drug medication and surgery. The very existence and constitution of the occupation lay in opposition to regular medical practices and theories. On the other hand, an occupation had to meet certain conditions if it was going to be in the race for a berth in tertiary education and for practitioner registration. Students had to obtain a 'proper' training in basic medical sciences and the representing association had to renounce claimancy to the throne that established medicine occupied.

The Webb committee made clear (1977, 128-129) that chiropractic and osteopathy should not be 'given legal recognition in any form that would imply that they were alternative health systems'. Nothing in the legislative definitions of chiropractic and osteopathy was to 'include and imply the principle of an alternative healing system which the Committee rejects'.

Chiropractors got the message: they played down claims that their medicine was an alternative — or, at least, a *complete* alternative — to orthodox medicine.[14] The VIC committee that decided to recommend placing the course at Phillip reported that:

the now clearly dominant perception of chiropractors [is] that their profession is one element in the spectrum of health services, not an alternative service; the official policy of the ACA regarding the place of chiropractic in the health care field reads: 'The ACA in no way claims or implies that chiropractic is an alternative total health care system in opposition to medicine. It sees chiropractic care as an alternative therapeutic measure in specific cases, but being part of the total health care system'.[15]

Again, the Webb committee (1977: 170) recommended the establishment of a bachelor degree of at least four years full-time study as the basic course of training. In 1977 a sub-committee of the VIC's academic committee in health sciences had said that a four-year course would be adequate to meet the aims envisaged and 'It is felt that the proposal [from PIT and the ICC] . . . for a five-year course could lead to an alternative medical course'.[16] At the start of 1978 the academic committee in health sciences commented:

A five year course as proposed by the Preston Institute is unnecessarily long, and could lead to a type of training which might be regarded as an alternative to medical training; this appeared to be in line with the philosophies of the American schools of Chiropractic, and the Academic Committee was not in sympathy with these philosophies.[17]

The chiropractors had to knuckle-under if they wanted accreditation. They did so by dropping their double-degree proposal which ran along the same lines as the orthodox medical combination of Bachelor of Medicine and Bachelor of Surgery (M.B., B.S.), by reducing the length of the course to four-and-a-half years and by creating a further six-month field practice requirement.

Chiropractors and osteopaths held that their occupations had become 'mainstream' health professions, as demonstrated by the institution of recognised higher education courses and practitioner registration. In the past, patients went directly to them because they had set up outside the system — they were, literally, alternative sources of assistance. They still might do so but primary contact was now justified by a collaborative relation: Phillip students were told that they were being trained to act as portals of entry to the Australian health care system.

The official position now was that chiropractic and osteopathy were not alternatives at all. Only their enemies called them that. In answer to renewed criticisms along these lines by the AMA (1992), the federal chiropractic association maintained that: 'Consistent with the desired co-operative health team approach, chiropractic does not perceive nor promote the profession as an alternative to conventional medicine' (CAA 1993: VII). While the advance of chiropractic:

> had not been accomplished without continuing resistance from conservative elements within its ranks (as the AMA should well understand), the profession proudly proclaims to have undertaken a paradigm shift enabling its principles and practice to conform with current scientific knowledge (1993, 7).

As Hobsbawm observed (1965: 11), 'In practice, every man who is not a Dr. Pangloss and every social movement undergoes the pull of both reformism and revolutionism, and with varying strengths and degrees at different times'. Chiropractors and osteopaths (and more recently, traditional acupuncturists) have been pulled toward internal reform by their desire to obtain legitimacy. Having met the externally imposed conditions for its allowance, especially by renouncing claims to be alternative medical systems, representatives of the occupations and many of the members then made the chiropractic radicals of old into 'conservative elements'.

One can well ask how legitimacy comes to be desired in the first place. The adherency of many practitioners in all three occupations seems to have shifted in familiar ways: from sharp opposition to the medical establishment to co-existence or even convergence. At the same time, chiropractic, osteopathy and traditional acupuncture continue to be repudiated by orthodox medical and physiotherapy associations. Teaching schools are pulled toward tightened controls on staff and student actions in order to defend the occupations against charges of disreputability. Their forms of regulative association also seem to have altered in familiar ways.

Many attempts have been made to 'locate' the so-called alternative, irregular, fringe or unorthodox medicines, that is, to fit them into a system of classification by reference to typical beliefs and practices. Very often, a religious analogy is pressed into service, or even literalised (as in Illich, 1975; 1977) so that 'the established church of medicine' takes on all the disabilities formerly belonging to Rome. Equally, religious and medical heterodoxy are likened — disparagingly when alternative medicines are called sects and cults.

Nevertheless, there are at least four grounds for drawing on the literature about religious groups for the study of medicines: (i) in each field a common purpose is met by discrete formations with comparable structures; (ii) historical relations between religious groups bear resemblance to those between medical groups; (iii) successful religious and medical groups appear to pass through similar organisational stages; (iv) the exponents pursue social betterment through redemptive measures (whether spiritual, physical or both). In what follows, the emphasis is on understanding the alternatives as collectivities offering medical services, not on making them into species of or substitutes for religion.

A religious application of the contrastive approach is found in Troeltsch's *The Social Teachings of the Christian Churches* (1931). He obtained his distinction between types of social organisation of the Christian idea from Weber (for his development of three pure types of legitimated domination, see *Economy and Society*, 1978, 215-216). Troeltsch set a mediaeval church-type against the emergent sect-type:

> The Church is that type of organisation which is overwhelmingly conservative, which to a certain extent accepts the secular order, and dominates the masses; in principle, therefore, it is universal, i.e. it desires to cover the whole of humanity. The sects, on the other hand, are comparatively small groups; they aspire after personal inward perfection, and they aim at a direct personal fellowship between the members of each group. From the very beginning, therefore, they are forced to organise themselves in small groups, and to renounce the idea of dominating the world (Troeltsch, 1931, 331).

The fully developed church utilised the state and the ruling classes, 'weave[d] these elements into her own life', and hence was an integral part of the existing social order, both stabilising and determining it. The church thereby became dependent on the upper classes and upon their development. On the other hand, the sects were connected to the lower classes (or at least with those social elements which were opposed to the state and to society): 'they work upwards from below, and not downwards from above' (p. 331). The church had 'this institutional principle of an objective organism', compared to which 'the sect is a voluntary community whose members join it of their own free will . . . an individual is not born into a sect; he enters it on the basis of conscious conversion' (p. 339).

Troeltsch established the church and sect as organisational forms but he did not account for the variety of sects, their internal contentions, and the changes each enduring religious group underwent over its history. Since the types appeared in different degree in all religious formations, an immediate problem was that Troeltsch 'thereby raised the question of quantitative proportion, and he was forced to deal with individual religious formations as though he were making a chemical analysis' (Antoni, 1962, 63-64). His typification, like so many others to follow, 'had the monotony of a classificatory exposition which lacked any trace of dialectical development' (p. 64). Absent was 'the negative moment, the insufficiency which translates itself into the painful need for and progression towards the new'.

H.P. Becker constructed a more elaborate scheme which overcame at least some of these shortcomings. He utilised the concept of secularisation (as developed by Tönnies, Durkheim and Malinowski, amongst others) and Weber's ideal types, to yield the analytic device of the isolated sacred society and the accessible secular society as 'methodological termini' (1932, 138). His typology was a scientific abstraction, as in the world of the theoretical physicist where irregularities were banished and the 'conscious fictions' of ideal form prevailed. The virtue of the points of reference established by marginal types was that they gave 'the determining orientation for the formulation of the results attained by empirical study' (p. 140). As Becker made clear, the accessible secular society was the 'methodological antithesis' of the isolated sacred (p. 142). The travel of the personality, activity or society in question was less clear, though Becker spoke of it as a process and usually in the direction of secularisation. He intended a transitional but overlaid sequence, as in his example of the marginal man (a term introduced by Robert Park in 1928) as:

> a human being controlled in part by character-attitudes deriving from an isolated sacred society, and in part differentiated and individuated by the influence of an accessible secular society, but not assimilated to those portions of that society (empirically speaking) in which attitudes deriving from isolated sacred societies prevail (H. P. Becker, 1932, 279).

In Becker's eventual typological sequence (cult — sect — denomination — ecclesia), political and economic institutions were closely interwoven with religious groupings (1956, 328-358). The appearance of cults was an index of advancing secularisation. They were frequently the first phases of sects, which 'in turn may be the point from which either a denomination or an ecclesia may grow' (p. 351). As a type, prophets stood in opposition to ecclesiastical priests and appeared in conjunction with cults and sects. They had a sense of mission and proclaimed a new message or, more frequently, attempted to revive an old religious teaching:

> In the technical sense of the term, they are often reactionary radicals, men who wish to go back to the past, and are therefore reactionary in that sense, but who wish to go back by digging down to the root of things, and are therefore radical in that sense (p. 353).

Religious mystics, many of them great cult leaders or models of sect religion, were somewhat withdrawn from contact with fellow human beings, communing with a spirit, a deity, 'with perhaps even something so vague as the totality of things, the All, the Whole' which could also be a focal point for cult recruitment (p. 355). The worshipper had a sense of merging in an all-inclusive whole, 'in an all-pervading reciprocity, a sense, in Chinese terms, of being at one with the Tao, of knowing the way, of being identified with the cosmos, the way of things' (p. 356).

Roth's study of United States and German natural health movements provides the outstanding example of the medical application of this schematisation. He used an extended metaphor to show how natural health groups follow the organisational sequence of religious movements:

> In terms of the revolutionary-reform dichotomy or the sect-church dichotomy the early stage of a movement is likely to be more revolutionary or sect-like and become less so as the sect progresses. With growing success, size, and generational change, they move towards compromise with establishment mores and greater acceptance of their social environment (Roth, 1977, 114).

Earlier chiropractic adherents were 'part of a mission following a prophet' (p. 118). They underwent some conversion experience which led to their acceptance of chiropractic and gave them a desire to follow this calling. But with growth, a greater number of those entering the field did so to earn a living and they were concerned with 'holding their own against the competition and with expanding their scope of practice if possible'. If that meant looking more like regular doctors and doing the things doctors did, then 'so be it':

> The organisational question becomes not 'how can we hold to the doctrine of our founder,' but 'how can we expand the career opportunities of our members.' And this means giving the clients what they want even if it requires many doctor-like activities. It means pursuing legislative lobbying to permit a broader scope of practice, that is, entering medical territory. It means moving into new areas (such as nutrition) not forbidden by law. It means working on prepayment, insurance, and government support schemes to improve their competitive position. Some members (the 'straights') disapprove of these changes, but if the organisation continues to grow, those favoring change (the 'mixers') will win out unless dominant forces (for example, very restrictive laws limiting chiropractic practices) prevent it. The straights can preserve their purity by seceding from the larger body, perhaps claiming that they are the original organisation and the mixers are the schismatics (p. 118).

Save for the extremity of revolutionary, millenarian, or certain isolated utopian communities, Roth said that membership of a social movement was not, typically, an all or nothing matter (p. 54). More frequently, those with some sympathy for the goals and activities of the movement were 'mixers' of some kind and degree. They lived in the larger society which did not accept or might not even know about the goals of the movement — which led to compromising behaviour:

> Thus, we should pay attention not only to who is favorable to the goals and activities of a given movement or movement organization; to who its leaders and followers are and to how they behave; but perhaps more importantly, the patterns of compromise and to the structural and interactional conditions that produce this behaviour (p. 55).

On Roth's account, then, successful religious and natural health groups travelled along an identical typological path: from the early or sect-like stage where the message was pure, the rejection of the extant order was clear-cut, and the aim was to obtain converts rather than to secure general endorsement, through the next stage, involving various sorts of compromise with the original doctrine, conflict over direction and the maintenance of purity, and a shift in emphasis to the protection of gains already won, to the end-state of being the establishment, being absorbed by or becoming a specialty within it, or petering out (pp. 114-122).

That medicines like chiropractic, osteopathy and traditional acupuncture follow a natural history of secularising progression from cult to church is not so evident. The early-middle-late categorisation (itself a version of the lower-middle-upper slots so endlessly applied to disaggregate all manner of social formations, hierarchies, and organisational lives) was meant to convey a patterned historical passage. The in-between condition then demanded its own resolution — by a social law of the excluded middle, as it were — either by the demise of the movement or by its onwards passage to establishment assimilation. The other inevitability was that dissidents would coalesce into fragments, detach from the establishment and return to the sect condition.

Everything can be fitted into and can serve to confirm this template because all the possibilities are allowed. A movement ceases to be successful when it does not progress, and vice versa. If a medicine endures but stays in much the same organisational condition, then attention is directed to factors inhibiting its alteration: what has to be explained is why this one medicine does not change, not why many do. But this immediately suggests the relativity of progression.

The 'natural' in natural history does not so much suggest the descriptive stage of new science as an unending cycle of occupational birth, contamination and fall, and reincarnation. The adjectival supplement raises as many problems for history as it does for medicine. Biological metaphors are frequent when analytical models lay out the internal unfolding of change, processes of organisational differentiation or, as Etzioni preferred (1966: 30-51), of epigenesis. In indicting historical theories based on biological analogies, Nisbet (1969: 250) noted that their emphasis in explaining change was on persons and purposes internal to the group and away from external factors. The same criticism holds for evolutionary interpretations. Collingwood (1963, 225) pointed out that the fallacy common to such views was 'the confusion between a natural process, in which the past dies in being replaced by the present, and an historical process, in which the past, so far as it is historically known, survives in the present'.

However important a critique of the principles and presumptions of classification may be, the systems in use are what counts here. We must remember that the protagonists of medicines often conceive their situation in religious *and* biological terms. The human organism is, after all, their subject and issues of doctrine and functional interrelation loom large. The designation of an occupational segment (or a whole medicine) as cultist indicates the desirability of taking steps to repudiate or extirpate it because it 'infects' the social body.

The assumption of occupational process, and of directional movement along the continuum between typological antitheses, was influential in the analyses of chiropractic by Wardwell, who commenced the sociological investigation of this occupation. In his earliest published work, based on his thesis, he developed the idea of a marginal social role out of Park's concept of the marginal man. The latter was marginal to two different — and, it should be added, incongruent — cultures. But Wardwell (1952: 340) used marginality, exemplified by the chiropractor (who, he said, was structurally comparable to the Negro), to refer to a single well-defined and imperfectly-institutionalised social role. He considered the chiropractic role would change since 'the dynamic nature of social systems implies incessant (though often minor) change in the definitions of social roles. Always some are in the process of becoming more fully institutionalised — others less so' (p. 348). His best guess then was that chiropractic would eventually merge in the medical mainstream.

Wardwell continued to hold to this analytical approach in subsequent publications. Using the medical profession 'as a touchstone', he arranged non-orthodox practitioners in a four-part classification according to such characteristics as their legal status and type of practice (1976, 62-64). While he did not explicitly state it, occupational groups were distinguished from each other by their distance from orthodox medicine. As a class, Wardwell referred to the unorthodox as irregular or cultist practitioners, and they were also described as being distinguished from orthodoxy along 'different dimensions of deviation', namely according to: the place in therapy of religion, magic, or supernatural entities; the related but secularised emphasis on 'the psychic side of the psychosomatic equation'; and adherence to alternative scientific theories and philosophies about illness causation and appropriate therapy (1976, 62). Internal divisions were also explained by reference to orthodoxy, that is, the strength of opposition to it (pp. 65-66).

Wardwell gauged the likelihood of convergence by occupational proximity to or distance from orthodoxy. A religious practice, such as

Christian Science, shared nothing at all with orthodox medicine whereas chiropractic 'differs from medicine in this respect only in placing greater emphasis on the *vix medicatrix naturae*, the innate intelligence of the body that makes cures possible' (1976, 67-68). He said the most a religious sect could evolve into was a denomination or church, but a healing sect, 'such as homeopathy, osteopathy, or chiropractic has at least the theoretic capability of evolving into medical orthodoxy, which is what happened to homeopathy around the turn of the century and is happening today to osteopathy' (1976, 68).

Nearly thirty years after his first paper on chiropractic, and in the light of considerable legislative and educational gains, Wardwell considered one possibility to be that chiropractic might become a parallel and independent medical profession, with chiropractors 'even more the equals of physicians while continuing to emphasize their differences' (1980, 35). Chiropractic was helped to continue on its present course in this direction by declining internal rivalry. The 'negative trade-off' was that occupations escaped medical domination by claiming only a limited therapeutic place and by not attacking 'medicine's basic theories concerning the nature of disease or the physician's dominant role in treating systemic or life-threatening illnesses' (1980, 36). As Wardwell said: 'Chiropractors cannot have their cake and eat it too' (p. 36).

From the start, Wardwell took an evolutionary approach to change and this became explicit in his later papers. He said (1988, 186-187) that chiropractic had evolved to a high level of acceptance and was unlikely ever to become an ancillary profession. Chiropractic had become 'so focused on spinal manipulation and hence so limited in its range of therapies that it cannot follow the course of osteopathy in moving ever closer to the medical mainstream'. The parallel profession designation, probably the most fitting term for osteopathy, was still conceivable for chiropractic if it continued to elevate education and practice standards. Wardwell still allowed the possibility of chiropractic remaining a marginal profession, stigmatised for its dubious theory and unacceptable to orthodoxy: many chiropractors had so well adapted to marginality that they might find acceptance more difficult to endure (1988, 188). By now, Wardwell's most likely possibility was that chiropractic might end up as a limited medical profession like dentistry, podiatry, optometry or psychology. The main reason these professions had evolved in the way they had, Wardwell said, was that the interests of the limited profession were more compelling than the interests of the overlapping medical specialties 'in treating such troublesome but routine problems as myopia, psychoneuroses, corns, or toothaches' (1988, 189). In his most recent publication (1992) Wardwell continued to hold to the idea of the marginal chiropractic role and to the likelihood of a separate but limited future for the occupation.

Wardwell considered the straight-mixer split to be 'a prototypical example' of a division framed in terms of degrees of variation from orthodoxy, with the straights holding to maximal difference and the mixers attenuating it (1976, 66). However, 'the terms really describe the two ends of a continuum rather than two discrete groups of chiropractors; most fall somewhere in the middle between the two poles, and this has probably always been true of the profession, although rhetoric belied the facts' (1988, 185). 'Somewhere in the middle' covered a lot of differences without indicating where and how the majority lay in this undifferentiated ground.

Chiropractic was likely to end up as a creature of the scheme that Wardwell intended to account for it. Though licensed, the marginality of chiropractors had to do with their stigmatisation by established medical practitioners and their associations (Sternberg, 1969, 225-226) and was a case of political rather than social and psychological marginality (Wild, 1978, 43). Rosenthal (1981, 274) said that if chiropractic continued to be a marginal occupation then it did so despite having many of the institutionalised characteristics of non-marginal or mainstream occupations. He noted that government and public acceptance had not been sufficient to gain physician recognition for chiropractic as a mainstream health care occupation and in this sense it remained marginal. Rosenthal asked (p. 274): 'To what extent has chiropractic moved from marginal to mainstream (assuming it was correctly classified as marginal)? Which attributes are indicators of which pole on an imaginary continuum from marginal to mainstream?'. He concluded that chiropractic remained marginal, though to a much reduced degree: 'But the difference between what chiropractic was and what it is now may have less to do with matters internal to chiropractic and more to do with how political, legal, and sociological assessments of chiropractic have changed and are changing' (p. 283).

Coulter (1983, 44) maintained that Wardwell had introduced 'a series of conceptions and assumptions about chiropractic that have been repeated by numerous social scientists since, and which have very little, if any, empirical support'. The examples he cited from

Wardwell's papers might all have evidenced various aspects of chiropractic marginality (the kind of people likely to join the occupation, the type of patients likely to be attracted to it and the reasons for their support, the greater frequency of unacceptable practices, and the unpreparedness to reconsider occupational tenets). But Coulter said that many were confounded by the available studies, such as the Canadian one in which he participated (Kelner et al., 1980). His own later demographic analysis showed that chiropractic patients were not dissimilar to the population at large in education, occupation and income distributions (Coulter, 1989).

Australian survey findings also suggested that chiropractic and other alternative medicines were not marginal in at least some of the respects indicated by Wardwell. For example, he said the vast majority of patients originally consulted chiropractors as a court of last resort. This was not borne out by respondents to an attitude to chiropractic survey who said they received previous treatment from a variety of sources, including chiropractors (Sheehan, 1985, 38).

Again, Wardwell maintained there were indications that proportionate to the total population more patients came from the lower classes and fewer came from the upper-middle class. A survey of the patients of alternative practitioners found that they had higher levels of education than the population at large (Dixon, 1986, vol.1, 55).

These results do not so much controvert Wardwell's assertions as highlight the absence of support for some of his generalisations. It was difficult to imagine how others — such as his comment that chiropractors probably had proportionately more hypochondriac and psychoneurotic patients; that patients might derive neurotic gratification of sensual or masochistic needs from chiropractic treatment; and that chiropractors could express aggressive urges by vigorous adjustments, using patients as objects for the displacement of hostility — might be ascertained at all or, if they could be, how it might be established that chiropractors and their patients were different from the practitioners of other medicines and their patients in these respects. Nevertheless, some established medical practitioners still make similar generalisations.

Coulter also disputed the contention that chiropractic was a deviant medical system (as suggested, for example, by McCorkle (1961) and Cowie and Roebuck (1975)). He said chiropractic might justifiably be so considered if it gave theoretical or descriptive insights but not if the designation was no more than a labelling exercise. He maintained that, in fact, the labelling of certain groups by others as deviant helped to constitute the very deviance. Those who had adopted the labelling approach 'seldom applied this insight to their own behaviour' (Coulter, 1983, 45). It was one thing to note that some powerful groups (like established medicine) labelled others as deviant 'but a totally different thing to label that group as deviant. In the former we act as observers, in the latter as labelling authorities' (p. 46).

Coulter had a sound case but he did less than justice to Cowie and Roebuck's argument. Having cited examples of the public diminishment of chiropractic theory and efficacy by persuasive labelling groups, they said the statements illustrated that chiropractors endured a deviant or at least marginal role in the United States (1975, 4-7). Coulter asserted that the statements did no such thing: 'They establish only that, at the level of rhetoric, some groups say chiropractic is deviant, and nothing more and nothing less' (1983, 45). But they did do something more when the groups concerned were influential. As H. S. Becker noted (1963, 6), the judgment of deviance was itself a crucial part of the phenomenon. Coulter might have been upset about the addition of sociological fuel to the authoritative fire but Cowie and Roebuck were largely concerned to discover how a practising chiropractor dealt with his social situation. He was not merely the passive recipient of a deviant label but an active promoter of chiropractic with a highly supportive professional reference group. Indeed, he recognised and took pride in his deviant status for it announced his loyalty to a higher cause.

The point is that the leaders of associations representing registered medical practitioners say something about their own reputability by way of saying that others are, objectively, deviant, marginal, cultistic and so on. To adapt Durkheim's point about criminality (1964, 81), one ought not to say that alternative medical practitioners are reprehensible because they are deviant and marginal but rather that they are deviant and marginal because they are considered reprehensible. Likewise, alternative practitioners did not define the 'crimes' of established medicine but were themselves defined by the identification of them.

Individuals or groups are liable to become 'instances' of the type. Noting that differences existed between the eighteen alternative practitioners they surveyed, Cant and Calnan (1991, 48) said that so far as their perceptions of role were concerned, these therapists 'located themselves along a continuum that ranged from separate and alternative to complementary and to the least demanding position of "supplement"'. They did no such thing. Cant and Calnan located them, according to a classification of their opinions. Where people locate themselves is another matter.

A further difficulty with the continuum idea can be traced to what Austin, in the course of discussing opposing philosophical doctrines about perception, calls 'the deeply ingrained worship of tidy-looking dichotomies' (1962, 3). Unlikes are drawn together through the construction of spurious antitheses like orthodox and unorthodox, church and cult, regular and alternative. By concentrating on one of the pair, kinds and classes are established out of heterogeneous assortments. The affirmed term, 'orthodox', for example, takes whatever sense it has from its opposite and is what Austin calls a 'trouser-word' (pp. 15, 70). To adapt his argument about terms like 'direct' and 'real', a definite sense attaches to the assertion of orthodoxy only in the light of a specific way in which it might be, or might have been unorthodox — 'it is the *negative* use that wears the trousers'.

Using the ideas of Bernstein (1973, 1977) others have established typificatory grids in order to account for the independent operation of social controls. Separately, Whyte arrived at a similar conclusion (1984, 230-233). He had supposed that co-operation and conflict in the peasant community were to be seen as the mutually exclusive ends of a single continuum. But field data led him to speculate about a different assumption — that co-operation and conflict were two separate and unrelated dimensions. He was able to make a single point location for co-operation and conflict scores by using a quadrant approach:

Figure 2   Conflict and Co-operation in 12 Villages

Cooperation	low conflict and high cooperation 1	high conflict and high cooperation 2
	3 low conflict and low cooperation	4 high conflict and low cooperation

Whyte, 1984, 232).   conflict

When there is frequent medical conflict, it is easy to assume that there is no co-operation or that conflict and co-operation follow each other in bouts. However, alliances and disputes within medicines and between them are woven into each other. Co-operation becomes important when conflict is thought to impede progress or even to leave the way open for occupational destruction (because established medicine will capitalise on internal dissensions, for example). Unity is not so much an occupational principle as a justification for a particular course of action directed to the attainment of specified mutual benefits; and continued dispute is not precluded by its accomplishment. To the contrary, dispute can be institutionalised by the terms of a unification settlement. The four combinations of high and low conflict and collaboration are overlaid in any one alternative medicine at any particular time, depending on the occupational segments and issues concerned.

Quadrant typologies can be applied to all manner of social formations. A version was used by Robertson (1972) to trace changes in the Salvation Army:

Figure 3   Path of the Salvation Army

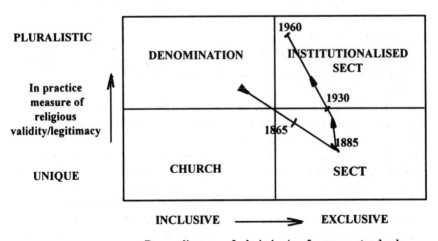

(Adapted from Robertson, 1970, 122, 128).

The institutionalised sect was introduced as a position between the sect and denominational types. According to Robertson (1972, 127), the Salvation Army had 'retained a sufficient number of its key pristine sectarian characteristics still to qualify in one sense as a sect, but has yet achieved a firm *modus vivendi* with the wider society'. He was not only referring to features of the Army (such as its membership becoming more 'respectable', more definitely lower-middle class) but also to changed social conditions: 'British society has become more tolerant of religious (and political) deviance since the crystallisation of the Army as a collectivity in the 1880s'. This raises an important point for all such typologies. Robertson charted the Army in relation to types of *religious* environment while allowing there was no constant relationship between the 'path' of a group and the wider society, for the latter itself changed. He emphasised that his typology was made in reference to a societal context (the 'position' of the Army would be different in another society where there was less tolerance of religious deviance).

In other words, typologies are built on shifting sands and the crucial question concerns the relationship between a group and various societal formations, ranging from those immediately impinging on the group to the most general social conditions. In a note, Robertson said this about his diagram:

> There are two extreme alternatives in interpreting this sequence. We can either view the Army as changing within a constant environment or the environment changing whilst the Salvation Army has 'stood still'. Empirically the sequence is a complex outcome of the interplay between the two factors. This general problem of analysis is a relatively uncharted, but also highly important one (Robertson, 1972, 146 note. 49).

To translate Robertson's example, chiropractic, osteopathy and traditional acupuncture might be considered in a health occupational typology utilising the same axes, namely measures of (i) the closed or open nature of admission and performance requirements (exclusive — inclusive); and (ii) the extent of in-practice concessions made about the acceptability and validity of other medicines (unique — pluralistic). Australian chiropractic and osteopathy commenced by being inclusive and unique. After the introduction of registration and government-supported higher education, they became exclusive and increasingly pluralistic. However, these indicative generalisations are relative to other forms of medical organisation and there is considerable internal divergence. Over the same period many other Australian health occupations also have become more exclusive and pluralistic.

Traditional acupuncture is rather different. In Australia, teaching and occupational groups associated with this medicine were at first inclusive and pluralistic. They became differentiated with the institution of private accreditation bodies and the extension of course requirements. Some (like the one studied here) have shifted toward exclusivity and uniqueness insofar as their relations with other traditional acupuncture organisations are concerned. Overall, however, the traditional acupuncture colleges are still more inclusive and rather less pluralistic than are registered occupations with courses in official tertiary institutions.

Robertson concluded that owing to its authoritarian military structure the Salvation Army had been 'relatively successful in maintaining the fairly tight-knit *epistemic communalism* of a religious sect' (1972, 127). It had established for itself an 'institutional slot' in British society and the one critical factor that had saved it from dissolution or absorption in another body was its relatively complex bureaucratic structure. These organisational considerations were only partly allowed for in his dimensions of membership principle and the in-practice preparedness of leaders to cede legitimacy and validity to other religious groups. While retaining the idea that successful groups exhibit complex structures of authority and membership differentiation, we need to understand changes to the principles of association and their relation to external social controls – the measures that Bernstein originally proposed in his classification and frame scheme.

Douglas took up Bernstein's ideas, first for the analysis of ritual (in *Natural Symbols*, 1973) and later for the grand enterprise of drawing together individual and group behaviour (in *Cultural Bias*, 1978). She replaced Bernstein's classification and frame with grid and group (1973, 82-85). Grid was the social dimension of shared or public classifications, whose influence ranged from weak (when private conceptions were ascendant) to strong (when societal controls were pervasive). Group referred to another and related sort of pressure – that put on the individual by positional associations, for example, in the family. Grid was the dimension or measure of individuation and group of social incorporation (1978, 7).

The interrelation of these dimensions was held to establish the framework for institutional life. The virtue claimed for the analysis was that it 'treats the experiencing subject as the subject choosing' and that 'each basic principle, the value of the group, the value of the individual, is the point of reference that justifies action of a potentially generative kind' (1978, 13). Another advantage was that the elaboration of group boundaries and the articulation of control structures were distinguished. Neither was seen as an inevitable process, though social pressures on the group might be considerable.

An example of the application of grid/group analysis will be considered. Rayner (1986) used group in the above way to indicate the degree of incorporation of the individual in a social unit (his case being a small British Trotskyist party). Grid referred to the nature of the interactions within the unit, that is, to the constraining rules bearing on the members of any social grouping (1986, 48):

Figure 4   Organisational Change: the International Socialists/Socialist Workers' Party

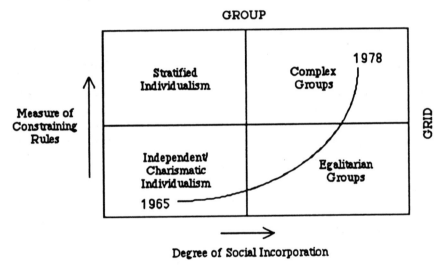

Degree of Social Incorporation

(adapted from Rayner, 1986, 49,62).

Over some ten years, the party shifted from being an open and egalitarian voluntary association (weak in group and grid) to one with a clearly demarcated membership and routinised authority structure (strong in group and grid). Along the way there were mass departures, factional suppressions and purges. Rayner made the following points: (i) the routinisation of authority in voluntary groups did not involve the gradual accumulation of rules that promoted internal inequality — instead, the construction of a strong group boundary was a necessary condition for the ultimate imposition of a complex organisational hierarchy; (ii) the transformation from loose-knit association (the alliance of diverse views where it was supposed that the opinion of each person carried the same weight) to solidaristic group (the social incorporation of participants) depended on a shared understanding of being apart from the wider society: 'Solidarity in the face of a common enemy is a credible value to charismatic individualists' (p. 63); (iii) on the other hand, the adoption of a hierarchical style characteristic of the world that threatened group members was in direct contradiction to their beginning expectations and future hopes; (iv) the routinisation of authority was not the inevitable product of irresistible forces (as Weber maintained, 1978, 246-254) but 'a conscious strategy, instigated by leaders wishing to formalise a voluntary association into a complex organisation' (p. 65); (v) nor was the change gradual and evolutionary — there could be quite rapid group transformations.

Alternative medicines also commence with bands of like-minded enthusiasts and minimal organisation. As representatives of other powerful groups come to discredit them and to attempt their suppression, they are subjected to formidable external constraints and antagonisms. In this situation, the leaders of alternative medical groups consolidate their hold over members and act strongly to define group boundaries, such as the style and range of acceptable training requirements and practice, and to solidify membership allegiance to standardised group values. The plethora of occupational associations and colleges does not just spring from the air: they frequently result from internal disputes over such boundary-controlling attempts on the part of leaders. Some leave the group while others persist in factions upholding their conceptions of group worth. These dissidents are removed when leaders establish that they have breached collegial requirements. Later we will find that members could be attacked for personal failings (for being too fanatical, not telling the truth, not actively participating) which effectively classified them as outsiders and so authorised their exclusion.

In its outward relations, a medicine relies on that systematic body of theory and skilled application which adherents claim to be singular to it. Abbott (1988, 18-20) wanted to pay more attention to the professional subject matter, to redress the concentration on the structure of power relations and professionalising processes. He considered the focus of a concept of professional development had to be the intimate relation of professional structure and culture to the work actually done. This development was bound up with interprofessional relations. Nothing could better demonstrate the latter point than the check to alternative medical enhancement schemes resulting from their not having the patronage of privileged medicines and indeed being subject to their outright antagonism.

The advancement of a medicine was one thing but its continued existence was another. Many practitioners of chiropractic, osteopathy and traditional acupuncture feared their occupations were in grave danger from established medicine and physiotherapy, not so much because of their attacks but because they were taking over the work. Strategically, this might be countered by: (i) drawing attention to the extensive education required for practice, the record of success with intractable conditions (i.e. where other medicines had failed), and special occupational capacities; (ii) marketing operations which kept the medicine and its achievements in sight and neutralised the dissemination of critical information (e.g. about the danger of occupational practices and their ineffectiveness) by competitors; (iii) staging the medical encounter by giving careful attention to the presentation of the clinic and the sequencing of patient events and interactions with staff (see Cowie and Roebuck's account, 1975, 47-105); and (iv) emphasising the public valuation of the medicine, the so-called 'demand', which constitutes a recognition of occupational expertise and effectiveness.

These activities were not unique to the alternatives, and practitioners did not engage in them to the same degree, but the sense of being in an underdog position gave impetus to the promotion of medical surfaces. There was, in addition, the question of the medical content. It was to be preserved from encroachment, but work was altered by the incorporation of technologies and by the standardisation of diagnostic measures and remedial techniques. What was the chiropractor, osteopath, and traditional acupuncturist to do with electronic products, such as the transcutaneous electrical stimulation devices being taken up by other competing medicines? Work was simplified and quickened by the use of such things, as it was by the extension of rule-based procedures. But mechanisation and routinisation could lead to increasing accessibility and even to the wholesale transfer of activities that previously demanded the skill of art and craft. Unlike the routinisation of authority, that of work carried the possibility of disenfranchising the professions, a prospect wrought by monopoly capitalism, according to Bravermann (1974, 403-409), and leading to the incorporation of professions as the intermediary layer in the polar class structure of capital and labour.

While the balance shifted from private practice to corporate and public sector employment, many professionals have retained a large measure of control of their knowledge and work. Willis (1983, 31-35) argued that technological innovations extended established medical dominance rather than reduced it. The increasing differentiation of medical labour was not driven by scientific and technical advances but by the social reinforcing of a vertical division which had established medicine delegating technical activities (e.g. radiography) and transferring mundane or time-consuming tasks to others in subordinate categories, such as nurses and aides.

Many alternative practitioners struggled to obtain a favoured place in this order *and* to keep up the separation of their work. The vulnerability of all medicines lay in their success. If their performances could be learned easily because occupational routinisation, including the publication of texts, made them accessible, then the very advancement of work led to its diffusion. An alternative medicine might take from established medicine — adopting its educational content, diagnostic categories and technical means — and be taken from in turn as other medicines assumed its practices.

The emphasis then turned back to work intangibles: the capacity to intuit bodily meanings and to invoke unspecifiable remedial arts. Hand-done work, the forte of chiropractic, osteopathy and traditional acupuncture, lent itself to such a bulwark. But it was not a case of one thing or the other. As Jamous and Peloille suggested (1970, 112), occupations were led in opposed directions by means of a production process that could be mastered and communicated through rules (what they called Technicality) and the means that escaped rules and 'at a given historical moment are attributed to virtualities of producers [Indetermination]'. Therefore the production process of any given occupation could be characterised by its Indetermination/Technicality ratio and 'the way in which the general balance of social forces, and the system of legitimacy which corresponds to it, uses and expresses this ratio in each historical situation' (p. 112). What counted in settling occupational certitudes and political actions were the contingencies of situation and the contradictions of purpose.

CONCLUSION

Movements can be classified in all manner of ways, by usual beliefs, behaviours, forms of association, authority structures, patterns of member exchange and by relations with other groups — those belonging, however contentiously, to the movement and those in the world-at-large, especially the dominant social formations that are at the centre of reform attention. Though it ought not be run too far, the religious analogy works best for medicine in this last sense.

The artifice of the category lies in its descriptive plausibility but makers are liable to be carried away by their analytical contrivances, converting their acts of selection into affirmations about the existence of identities and differences, and justifying their classes by claims about the suitability of assignments to them. On inspection, however, medicines and religions participate, to a greater or lesser extent, in all available types. They are imposed on phenomena as supposedly objective categories yet they formulate their own subject-matter. Even so, as Beckford says about new religions: 'The need for typologies and classifications is beyond doubt if we are to understand more about the social dynamics of these distinctive movements' (1985, 76). Other valuable understandings are to be found in the summaries of religious types provided by Hill (1973, ch. 4) and Wilson (1973, chs 1,2).

There is no particular frame that 'fits' the situation of chiropractic, osteopathy and traditional acupuncture and that can be used to account for their movement. The medicines changed, in the sense that their practitioners fought for and obtained advantages like higher education and registration. They became more organised. The occupational substance altered, not entirely or consistently, in the sense that the convictions and practices of a majority differed from those of a majority a decade before. All the same, practitioners still identified themselves with the medicines, still disputed with each other and still encountered antagonism in much the same way as they had always done.

These constancies were related, as will become plain in the following chapters.

Notes

1. The Preston director looked beyond chiropractic to an extended engagement in natural therapies for his college. He courted the osteopaths. Just before the critical meeting of the chiropractic course location committee of the Victoria Institute of Colleges, the AOA president asked whether Preston would be

prepared to set up a course advisory committee for the establishment of an undergraduate programme in osteopathy. The AOA member vigorously supported Preston at the VIC meeting. Shortly after it, the director confirmed that his college 'would be pleased to assist in every possible way to establish this programme'. See the account in O'Neill (1991b, 385-389).

2. 'Disciples have nearly always exercised a pernicious influence on the thought of him they call their master and who has often believed himself obliged to follow them . . . disciples expect their master to close the era of doubt by giving final solutions to all problems' (Sorel, 1961, 29).

3. 'Minutes of Chiropractors' Meeting', 15 August 1938, ACA archives.

4. Minutes, Annual General Meeting, Australian Chiropractors' Association, 14 September 1940, ACA archives.

5. Minutes, Executive, Australian Chiropractors' Association, 7 August 1941, ACA archives.

6. Minutes, Executive, Australian Chiropractors' Association, 7 August 1941, ACA archives.

7. 'Notes on meeting with UCA and naturopaths to discuss Registration legislation', 18 May 1977, SCO archives.

8. Handwritten notes of the meeting, n.d (October/November 1977), SCO archives.

9. Fawke, to the directors of the other colleges, 21 November 1977, SCO archives.

10. Letcher, PIT acting principal, to Blake, VIC council secretary, 25 November 1988, VIC archives.

11. Circular to ACA members, n.d. (November 1977), SCO archives.

12. Martin, S. Letter to the Editor, *A.C.A. News* 15, 5 (1988), p. 9.

13. 'Firstly, we believe that **registration of non-medical acupuncturists would amount to government sanction of a potentially dangerous treatment by lay people . . . if not properly carried out, acupuncture is potentially life-threatening'**. Emphasis in the original, 'The Australian Medical Acupuncture Society Submissions Re: National Acupuncture Register for Lay Acupuncturists', 1990.

14. For example, in the ACA's 'Submission on Chiropractic Course Siting to the Ad Hoc Committee on Chiropractic of the Victoria Institute of Colleges', December 1978. VIC archives.

15. Victoria Institute of Colleges. 'Ad Hoc Committee on Chiropractic Report', 8 January 1979, p. 5., VIC archives.

16. At a meeting on 12 December 1977 and recorded in the VIC paper, 'Chiropractic/Manipulative Therapy-Master Plan Proposals — Report of Subcommittee', 19 December 1977. VIC archives.

17. At a meeting on 9 February 1978 and recorded in the VIC paper, 'Chiropractic/Manipulative Therapy Education-Master Planning Recommendation', 10 February 1978, VIC archives.

IV

THE PHILOSOPHERS

How far is all their action intended to save chiropractic from others and themselves?

(Fifth year chiropractic student.)

B.J. HAD A SAYING . . .

Reggie Gold, an American who often visited Australia to spread the message, was the sort of backward-looking chiropractor the school despised. A Victorian parliamentary select committee (Ward, 1975, 61) had said of him:

> 'Mr. Gold was a chiropractic evangelist who, in the opinion of the Committee, would damage any profession with his oratory . . . Mr. Gold had a great emotional appeal and his approach to giving evidence was basically on the public relations technique of few facts but plenty of colorful presentation.'

The chiropractic and osteopathy school at Phillip quite agreed. For that matter, Reggie had a low opinion of the school. He told a meeting (well attended by its students) that the Palmers made their first major mistake when they increased their course from three to six months: 'The colleges started to teach more and more medicine and less and less chiropractic — the lower your vision the broader the scope!'

Reggie said chiropractors had sold their birthright to gain medical acceptance:

> You don't have to practise chiropractic the way they teach you. You don't have to be ashamed of it, you can be proud of it . . . No one will know you are a quack, except me — I'll *know* you are a quack! . . . Half your chiropractors in school try to drag you down into the gutter, telling you that you are no better than a physical therapist or an osteopath. Sometimes they merge the two. Your task at school is to get the piece of paper. You are being lied to day and night, you

are being told you can diagnose. You learn diagnosis out of text-books. The medical doctor does an internship, then he does a specialty. Are we, in ten minutes in a mickey mouse school going to diagnose everything? Don't kid yourself that you are doing people a favour when you practise wrong diagnosis. I think it shows more integrity when you say you don't do those things.

A student asked Reggie what sort of course he would teach. He replied, with the logic that marks those who countenance no piecemeal measures: 'How can I teach a course and get my people licensed? I couldn't. So I asked, why get them licensed?' He had set up a nine-month course but had cut it down to six months. Like Paracelsus (1990, 72), who wanted it known that the pillars of his medicine were philosophy, astronomy, alchemy and virtue, Reggie had clear ideas about what was important: 'The philosophy you learn in chiropractic college could be done in two weeks. Music, classical philosophy, astronomy, will be a better education for chiropractors than medical subjects'. At their school, students were forced to learn 'micro-minutiae' — out of date even as they learned it: 'The new science of Einstein, and carried on by Fritjof Capra, is coming around to the idea that Newtonian science is wrong'.

Reggie held that the capability to recover from any disease was inherent in the living body: 'B.J. said if you hit them in the arse with a shovel and kick them down a flight of stairs, *some* of them will get well. Now, this is *not* the technique of choice!'

To call themselves chiropractors, the one skill they had to have was finding the vertebral subluxation. A student asked what caused a subluxation. Reggie said: 'A failure of the body to adapt to some force, chemical, emotional, electrical as well as physical. The first cause is obstetricians. Obstetricians just *hate* nature!' How did he locate the vertebral subluxation?

Everything I do is philosophical. There is an innate awareness of every innate need. The body *knows* what it needs. My philosophy in chiropractic says the innate wisdom knows everything. Trust the bloody body. When the body needs an adjustment, don't you think it *knows* that? It does, but sometimes it needs a little help. It is the job of Innate Intelligence to adapt universal force to kinetic force.

Another student suggested that the graduates of short courses would only be technicians. 'Only a technician? That's just a way of pouring crap on a name! I found it so hard to get PIT students *up*. How do you do that when you know what you are doing for five years is garbage, crap?'

The fact that chiropractic was mandated as a primary care occupation did not mean the students *had* to extend their range of therapies. When chiropractors corrected the subluxation — 'not the one you see on x-rays, you can't see subluxations on x-rays' — they totally destroyed chiropractic practice because the patient went away thinking they were cured and never came back. That was the medical way: 'The worst thing we ever took from the medical profession was their bloody fees system!' Subluxations were always there. Reggie had only ever seen one patient who was subluxation-free; that did not mean the patient *was* free of subluxations, only that he could not find them. He argued for prevention. The time for chiropractic care was before one got disease. Subluxations had no symptoms: 'Sure, some of them hurt, most of them don't'. He favoured a maintenance plan where families signed up (at a fixed annual price) for regular vertebral subluxation checks and adjustments.

Chiropractors had to have a vision, a fire, to understand their heritage and to be proud of it:

> Most of us are desperately in need of approval . . . Chiropractors are a minority and that's the problem. Minorities get picked on. I met a black chiropractor in Kansas and he said, you know, being black and being a chiropractor is like being black twice.

Thousands of people died every day because no-one had told them about chiropractic. How wonderful it was to be free of subluxations! That was the vision they should never lose: 'I don't want politicians with one hand on the red phone and the other on the death button when they are subluxated!'

Chiropractors had a mission. Reggie had practised seven days a week: 'I don't see how you can sit around there [in church] when there are subluxated kids outside without treatment. Are you going to crap around there on Sunday when there's a job to be done?'

At the end of his three hour talk, Molloy, a local chiropractor, thanked Reggie on behalf of the Chiropractic Society of Australia (CSA). The event had not been conducted at the school — it would not permit such 'extremists' on the campus. But the audience was transfixed by the singleness of Gold's purpose and by his remarkable oratory. A third year student said to me afterwards: 'You see, we are *up* there and we'll just go back into the college and it will drag us down again'. Others nodded agreement. The previous year they had complained about the absence of philosophy and of a 'positive attitude' in the course. Many did not see the point in what they were doing at the school. They said the basic sciences — chemistry, biochemistry, microbiology — were not integrated into their studies. The diagnostic sciences were never practised — Reggie was correct about that. All the time medicine said 'follow us and do this', but it would never admit chiropractors as equals. Reggie was also right about that. They just had to keep on in the school until they could get out and be *enthused* about the practice of chiropractic. It was hard going in the school but as Molloy said when he introduced Gold: 'Reggie had a saying — when you get to the end of your rope, tie a knot and hang on!'

THE CSA

The Chiropractic Society of Australia, founded in November 1985, was a late competitor in the associational stakes. In seeking Australasian Council on Chiropractic Education (ACCE) recognition for it, the foundation secretary, Molloy, wrote that the CSA had been formed after years of dissatisfaction with some aspects of the other two associations:

> The general feeling was that these associations spent a great deal of time and money in gaining benefits for the Chiropractor but failed to actively promote the purpose of Chiropractic. In many instances they even wasted time, energy and money on promoting disciplines other than Chiropractic, such as acupuncture and electrotherapy.[1]

Molloy believed the path taken by the ACA 'was veering away from the original concepts of Chiropractic'. In an earlier letter to the dean of the school, Molloy elaborated these shortcomings.[2] The establishment of modality committees and acupuncture committees within the ACA evidenced a trend away from the original philosophy as defined by D.D. and B.J. Palmer; this led to internal friction between opposing forces wishing to establish their 'brand' of chiropractic. The majority of ACA members made a healthy income out of chiropractic but were 'reticent about putting any of that income back into the publicising of the profession's approach towards health care'. The CSA's 'main purpose' was to instigate and fund public education programmes: the ACA 'spent a great deal of time feathering the nests of the Chiropractor but not necessarily enhancing the benefits to the patient, or promoting Chiropractic'.

The CSA adhered to a strict interpretation of chiropractic, closely resembling that of the Sherman College of Straight Chiropractic in the United States (where, in earlier years, Gold had lectured in philosophy). The scope of member practice was restricted to (a) the location, identification and categorisation of vertebral subluxations; (b) their correction by adjustments; (c) patient and public education in chiropractic philosophy and principles; and, as the constitution had it, '(d) Nothing else'.[3]

School responses to the CSA were predictably negative. The dean told me that if he could, he would ban Molloy and his kind from visiting the school to talk to students. He appears to have done so even before the formation of the CSA. In 1984 he told the commission on accreditation of the Australasian Council on Chiropractic Education (ACCE) that:

> Concern has been expressed on the part of certain members of staff over possible cultistic concepts which may have crept into the teaching of chiropractic science. A plan of action to deal with this matter is being formulated.[4]

Six months later, student class representatives were told that 'certain lecturers would not be allowed on campus'.[5]

MOLLOY'S ODYSSEY

Given the need to protect students from outside influence, members of the CSA came from an unlikely source. The initial Australian members were Phillip graduates, with a minority of North American graduates.[6] Molloy was amongst the first group of students to enrol in the International College of Chiropractic course, and one of the inaugural graduates from it in May 1979.

Molloy told me that he was a 'big mixer' on graduation, knowing little about the philosophy of chiropractic. He went to Queensland early in 1980 and worked with a chiropractor called Charlton. Molloy and Charlton talked and argued a lot about philosophy. Later in the year, Molloy attended a seminar run by an American chiropractic group called Renaissance. He dated the beginning of his philosophical commitment to that experience.

Renaissance offered courses designed to help practitioners improve public and patient awareness of the chiropractic message. A Renaissance brochure spoke of a New Age consciousness evolving in chiropractic, resulting in a seminar with a world plan:

> This plan has as its goal the birth of the Magical Child: a child without subluxation, born free of the fear of becoming subluxated, into a society which is conducive to harmonious living with our environment, and eventually, the appearance of the Renaissance man and woman: a planet of unsubluxated people living within an unsubluxated social and environmental framework.[7]

The brochure depicted suffering humanity in decline through orthodox medicine, then passing upwards through mixing chiropractic until it reached the plateau of straight chiropractic, whereupon unsubluxated generations travelled across to enlightenment:

Figure 5   Renaissance Path to the New Age

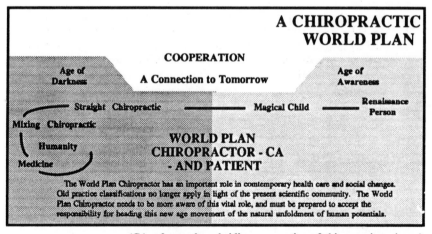

(CA refers to the subsidiary occupation of chiropractic assistant)

In the accompanying model talk for prospective patient information sessions, subluxations occurring during or shortly after birth were identified as the real cause of the human condition, 'robbing us of our innate potential for a very long, very healthy and very happy life'. The subluxation was, so the speak, the legacy of Adam. Yet an answer was at hand. The chiropractor cleared subluxations by adjusting, just as the sacrament of baptism cleansed the original sin.

A teacher called such ideas 'bio-theology, philosophical wanking', but they were an epiphany for Molloy. He said that in 1982 he spent $3 000 on books by B.J. Palmer. He was embarked on the contentious path of the reformer who is called (and is to become) a sectary for demanding adherence to the foundation creed.

Molloy attended the 1983 annual federal general meeting of the ACA as a Queensland representative, and said that meeting was the start of his real falling out with the association: 'What I was trying to do was to straighten up chiropractic'. He tabled a motion which said (as he recollected), 'We view with concern the direction chiropractic is heading with the mixing of modalities'. The debate was fiery and he was opposed by Victorian branch members. The motion was laid on the table. Nothing more happened about it until the Queensland branch met prior to the November 1984 meeting of the federal executive. Molloy raised the matter of his tabled motion and wanted to know what was to happen about it:

> Charlton is a representative [of the branch for the federal meeting] and he is doing a lot of yelling and shouting. A number of people were right into what I was doing. Keith [Charlton] comes from a very medical model. John Hinwood was federal vice-president of the ACA and he was right into what I was doing. That's when we started organising and setting up the Australian and New Zealand Straight Chiropractors' Association, ANZSCA, that is, the 'answer'.

Molloy said this group was established by early 1985. It had:

> A cellular division — apart from myself everyone else only knew two other members. No one would know who was in the organisation apart from me. It was undercover. If they knew who all the other members were they'd block it. The effect was to get as many of our members into [state and federal] executives across Australia to change it [the ACA] without their knowledge. If anyone racked off they couldn't blow it. Basically we'd get these people interested, rugby people often. [As a student Molloy had been active in establishing a college team to play rugby union — something of a deviant game in the state of Victoria.]

Molloy sold his Queensland practice (to a Sherman graduate) and after spending several months overseas visiting American colleges, he returned to Victoria to set up practice in Geelong, his home town. By early 1985, about the time that ANZSCA became active, Molloy had joined the Victorian executive of the ACA. He was soon in dispute with it.

The school was troubled. Its executive committee agreed that some alumni should meet with Molloy to express concern at some of the statements he had made about the school.[8] Molloy was instrumental in arranging for Dr Thom Gelardi, president of Sherman college, to visit Australia and wanted him to talk at the school. The dean said 'no way'. The executive decided that Gelardi would not be allowed to lecture on campus.[9] A month later, there was a report of Molloy presenting a lecture to third-year students at the invitation of a staff member.[10] Students were said to have complained about his philosophy and the chiropractic sciences department decided the class should be advised that Molloy had not been authorised to be on campus and that the school did not endorse what he had said. The dean reminded staff that 'no unauthorised guest lecturer may lecture on campus' and told them of the correct procedure, which involved getting approval from the appropriate head of department.[11]

A legend began to grow up about Molloy. A graduate remembered the incident as follows:

> When I was a student we had a temporary lecturer who got Terry in to talk to us. The powers-that-be were really mad about that! They told security he was not permitted in the school. He was banned from being there.

Whether true or not, it was generally believed that Molloy had been excluded from visiting the school and having contact with students (though no one told him so formally, then or later). A former staff member who was present when these events took place said that while the decision was to ban only an American who was out in Australia at the time (Gelardi), Molloy was associated with him in some way and he 'kind of got added to the list of people not to be given permission to speak to students'. There was no committee resolution to this effect but the school had taken another step towards enclosure and the regulation of staff and student actions. It had not always been thus: Molloy said that his class had watched a video of a talk by Gold on the first day of teaching in the new school.

Molloy and his group were being blocked. If they could not work clandestinely from within to achieve their ends then they would have to move from without and in plain sight. Molloy told me that Tremaine, another Phillip graduate, rang him and said: 'We have to have an open organisation, we must get the message out to the public'. On 24 August 1985, twenty-one chiropractors went to dinner at a seafood restaurant (they were in Sydney for a seminar) and decided to form the CSA to promote chiropractic. According to Molloy, the CSA did not start as a 'straights' organisation but very quickly became so. He said many pulled out when they saw the constitution and others came in but did not last.

The following month (September 1985) the message about the formation of the CSA was well and truly abroad. The ACA held its annual general meeting in New Zealand and Molloy was queried about the new body. One member asked Molloy whether the CSA was another name for the ANZSCA. Molloy told me he had answered that it was not. He was also asked whether this meant he was leaving the ACA (he was still on the Victorian branch executive). Of this time, Molloy said: 'A lot of people are coming across to the CSA, a lot wanting to be in both camps but pissed off with the ACA. A lot of fighting, a lot of things not going right.'

Molloy became totally disillusioned and resigned from everything: 'I'd had enough of hitting my head against the wall trying to get people to do something they didn't want to do. I thought I'll just go back and do what I want to do.' The withdrawal was short-lived. Tremaine rang him up again and said that he had just called Reggie Gold. Gold said he would come out to Australia. Molloy agreed to go to the inaugural general meeting of the CSA on 30 November 1985, which Gold addressed and over sixty chiropractors attended.[12] And then Molloy was involved again. He said he was asked to be president of the new body but refused in favour of being secretary, knowing that the secretary was the most powerful man in the organisation. Shortly before that meeting, the dean told the school executive that the CSA had been formed. In an understatement, the minutes reported that members noted this 'with some concern'.[13]

In January 1986 Molloy sought to address incoming students on behalf of the CSA. The dean was away at the time and Molloy was fobbed off until he returned.[14] When he did, Molloy was not refused but was asked to explain his organisation and its purposes and to indicate what he would like to convey to students. Letters were exchanged but Molloy never got approval. When I said to a teacher that it seemed the school did not want its students exposed to Molloy, he told me that the explanation he had heard given was that the school did not want Molloy associating his name with it, that is, being able to put down on his 'history' that he had lectured in the school.

The ban on Molloy continued to be effective. A teacher said that in 1988 he had been approached by a first-year student about having Molloy speak to the class. While not personally opposed, he suggested that the students arrange the talk off campus. As the teacher told me:

> The school line is something I have to acknowledge and accept and I do so because I think it is reasonable for the school to have a line. But I have my own views about what we are liable to forget — the worth and value of chiropractic and the criticisms that there are of medicine.

He and some other teachers privately disagreed with the 'line' and thought the school should be more flexible, more open. Molloy's separate account is instructive. He said that a first-year student had recently rung up and asked him to come out and talk to the class. He had told her that he was happy to do so but did not know whether he would be allowed on campus. Molloy rang a student contact of his and it was agreed that the best way to proceed was for an approach to be made to the teacher referred to above who was considered sympathetic to 'straights' thinking.

Molloy kept on pressing for access. He said that the alumni association (CAAPIT) had been discussing having some of their members talk to students. He had written to the president of the association about his preparedness to do so but she said that the dean had rejected him as a speaker 'because he could use for his political benefit the statement that he lectured to students of PIT'.

Molloy took some comfort from a letter he had received from the dean at the end of his first year as a student. The dean had congratulated Molloy on his creditable performance. The college was proud of him and wished him well in his future studies. In a postscript the dean said:

> The deficiency in Philosophy is of a minor nature requiring some additional work, and does not delay your promotion to the second year. However, it will have to be corrected at the earliest date possible, and no later than March 15th, 1977.[15]

Molloy certainly had done that.

THE LIABILITY OF HERETICS

Like an itinerant Beghard of northern Europe in the fourteenth century, Gold wandered the world spreading a version of the gospel, to the dismay of the local ecclesiastical authorities. Such people could be captured and put to the torch in mediaeval times, an option (to judge from the strength of their reactions to Gold and his kind) that many chiropractors would like to have retained. A student contemporary of Molloy said:

> The profession has a love/hate relation with Terry. He presents stuff so that it appears he is attacking them. As a group, if they had their way, if he was being burned at the stake they would be throwing on the kindling. He asks all these good questions such as, 'but *why* are you doing it?' Terry is in and out of our organisations, firing arrows as we go past.

Keeping Gold (and Molloy) out of the school was justified by saying that chiropractic got a bad name from their promulgation of unscientific, cultistic nonsense. The hard-won status of chiropractic was jeopardised by them, not because their ideas were potent and others might easily be converted to the same way of thinking (I never heard that given as a reason) but because the cultists manufactured and handed over ammunition to the opposition. There was this sense of disloyalty to chiropractic in being a 'straight'; of assisting in its destruction by playing into the hands of the enemy, possibly even of being frenzied enough to do so with malice. How could it be that some of those carefully selected and educated graduates of the school could go into Reggie Gold's camp? That the school might have given rise to such a liability was unthinkable: since no-one of right mind could possibly accept the 'straights' philosophy, those who had fallen in with it must have turned fanatical.

There was another reason for establishment ire. Prophetic messengers for original truths tread a thin line between constructive criticism and heresy. The difference has less to do with gradations in the content of belief than with an unpreparedness to be publicly submissive to authority. Gold was no St. Francis. He not only preached a return to chiropractic fundamentals but also set up schools of spinology in opposition. After sitting next to Gold at a 1985 Queensland chiropractors' Christmas banquet, Charlton (Molloy's former mentor during field work) told his colleagues:

I asked him about his school — he said there were now four — one, his, in Philadelphia, one started in San Francisco by one of his graduates, one in Valencia, Spain, and one in Lima, Peru. He said he is the only teacher in his school and that fifteen students attend 9 a.m. to 1 p.m. for one year. They then practise the detection and elimination of vertebral subluxation. He hopes these schools will proliferate around the world.

I enquired about curriculum, and he said that there was a great deal of philosophy, and adjusting the spine (he says the pelvis does not fall within the ambit of a 'straight' philosophy). There is no science (in the generic sense) taught, nor diagnosis or x-ray. He says that these are unnecessary.[16]

As Gold told Charlton, the chiropractic profession had abandoned its true vocation of relieving subluxation. Gold's message and the literature of the Renaissance group demonstrate how much the straights had in common with Christian millenarian movements. A new age for humanity would be ushered in once subluxations were identified and adjusted. Subluxations were not part of the divine ordination but caused by humans. Their origin was made plain in a poster commonly seen in straights clinics: it showed the hands of a doctor twisting an infant head (the face contorted with pain) at the moment of birth.

Cohn (1970, 13) used millennarianism to label a particular type of salvationary belief which was:

(a) collective, in the sense that it is to be enjoyed by the faithful as a collectivity;

(b) terrestrial, in the sense that it is to be realised on this earth and not in some other-worldly heaven;

(c) imminent, in the sense that it is to come both soon and suddenly;

(d) total, in the sense that it is utterly to transform life on earth, so that the new dispensation will be no mere improvement on the present but perfection itself;

(e) miraculous, in the sense that it is to be accomplished by, or with the help of, supernatural agencies.

Even the last might apply to the subluxation, for its adjustment enabled the Innate to express Universal Intelligence, the therapist being merely a facilitating agent.

Straight chiropractic runs close to the manipulationist type (no pun intended!) in Wilson's (1973) compilation of varieties of new religious (but not specifically Christian) movements. Rather than classifying them in terms of their statements of mission or redeeming purpose, Wilson associated the range of sectarian orientations with prevailing conditions in the wider society. Thus, sects were understood as dependent on prevailing circumstances, as 'responses to the world'. They do not remain fixed but 'mutate' through the attenuation of original value commitments. According to Wilson:

> No less than other responses this [manipulationist] orientation is concerned to provide timeless happiness for man . . . Whatever the ideologies of manipulationist movements may be, this response is very much related to every-day well-being, and this well-being may be vouchsafed by learning universal principles concerning man and the world which will explain evil away. This conception of salvation is neither other-worldly nor transcendental. It is the scarce goods of the world — health, wealth, longevity, happiness, success, high status — which constitute the saved condition (1973, 24).

Since the manipulationist sect 'offers both objective achievement and psychic reassurance in a world in which the direct reassurances of participation in community life have been weakened' (Wilson, 1973, 41), it is likely to arise in highly individuated and achievement-oriented societies. Hill has noted that such typical features of new religion (which he summarises) resonate with 'the life experiences of mobile, educated individuals in a modern society' and suggest that 'We should therefore expect to find a significant and growing proportion of the populations of western societies having some contact with, or at the very least knowledge of the area of new religions and — what I shall argue is a closely related phenomenon — complementary therapies' (1992, 224-225). Hill later remarks that 'Manipulationists have often been characterized as syncretistic, combining the insights of modern science with their own special gnosis to produce a novel amalgam, so that in their therapeutic mode they should be evident on the fringes of orthodox medicine' (1993: 152-153). He goes on to say that the usual loose-knit, fluid form of organisation of manipulationist groups is to be seen amongst New Zealand complementary therapies.

Similarly, if new religious movements are considered as 'distinctive sets of social relationships' (Beckford, 1985, 77) and characterised by their 'modes of insertion' in their societies then straight chiropractic is like them in being distinguished by its emphasis on revitalising and transforming the secular world. In the other direction, 'The position of NRMs (New Religious Movements) committed to revitalization is therefore similar to that of many non-religious voluntary association in advanced democratic polities' (Beckford, 1985, 87).

All the same, straight chiropractors have much in common with old-style sectaries. Molloy's association began as a conventicle but then spread its message outwards to the people. Early chiropractic — all that B.J. Palmer stood for — figured large with the CSA, as the early church did for the sects. And there was a latter-day Elijah. Cohn's remarks (1970, 261) about John of Leyden, the Anabaptist leader of a 16th century Münster uprising, are apt: 'For here, as so often — as in the case of "the Master of Hungary" and many another in the Middle Ages and indeed at all times — the messianic leader was to be the stranger, the man from the periphery.' Like D.D. Palmer, Gold was the charismatic loner, the travelling inspirational source. B.J. Palmer had said (1979, 338):

> As Chiropractors, we recognise our duty to be adjusters of the CAUSE of sickness, drunkenness, and poorness. We have connecting link between God and man — that knowledge of cause supplies necessity.

Like him, Gold and his deductive kind were armed with certitude.

One form of Marxist analysis led to a similar conclusion. Althusser (1977, 13) said that Marx's fundamental discovery was in danger of being forsaken by those who adjusted theoretical concepts in the light of the times. Equally, Gold, Molloy and like-minded advocates of original chiropractic thinking were at pains to reverse a shift toward convergence. The health message had been obscured and degraded by compromise. It had to be made pure and absolute again.

STAFF AND STUDENT REACTION

Attempts to keep out the likes of Gold and Molloy, and the advocates of embracing diagnostic and technique systems like SOT (Sacro-Occipital Technique) and AK (Applied Kinesiology), would seem excessive only to those who do not have the experience of prejudicial dealings. Chiropractors announced their reputability — their having joined the mainstream, being members of the health care team — but they continued to be made into strangers and kept apart. Any association of the school with 'untenable' beliefs and practices was fuel to the fire of this antagonism. Consider the position of teachers who found, for them, nonsensical assertions in material circulated in the school. One took exception to an article in a SOT newsletter which, amongst other things, advised the practitioner (in capitals) to

> MAKE A HEALING CIRCLE OF THE RIGHT HAND THUMB AND INDEX FINGER AND PLACE OVER THE CONCERNED ACETABULAR FOR 30 SECONDS. CONCEPTUALLY CONCENTRATE THE TISSUES MELDING TOGETHER WITH THE POWER OF THE HAND ENERGY SPECTRUMS.[17]

The teacher castigated the whole approach as unscientific.[18] His other concern was that, at the request of the SOT association, the school had allowed its newsletters to be left at the front desk for students to pick up:

> As often happens, these types of publications are left lying in public areas such as cafeterias. The newsletter then becomes, directly or indirectly, available to students and academics of any discipline at Phillip Institute. These individuals request clarification and those of us who work towards a rational groundwork for chiropractic treatment, whether empirical or proven in research, must explain to our fellow professionals outside chiropractic how this type of irrational explanation and treatment is also considered part of chiropractic . . .

> I feel that it is our responsibility as professionals to uphold the credibility of our profession. Discussion of treatments in such an unprofessional manner as in the present (SOTO A/sia Ltd.) Newsletter can only cause a loss of esteem from those outside the profession and a source of anger and embarassment to those of us dedicated to the improvement of the chiropractic profession.

Other staff were less concerned about barricading the school's reputation. Molloy and the like *were* chiropractors. Many students came into contact with them at outside seminars. It was better to expose students to the variety of opinion in the profession. They would, at any rate, arrive at stances and so a spirit of critical and informed debate should be promoted. That was the job of tertiary institutions.

Whether people like Molloy should or should not be allowed into the school was discussed *as if* it were a singular question but views on the matter went along with and gave expression to attitudes about profession and school. Teachers who were disaffected with the profession supported controls. They were school insiders, and outsiders to the profession: the school had to be protected from its worst professional self. Another teacher who took exception to the 'cultistic nonsense' of SOT gave as example a claimed '30 second adjustment to eliminate Candidiasis'.[19] He told me: 'When you write your thesis you should make clear that not all chiropractic is a lunatic fringe. *Every* profession has its lunatic fringe, except that our lunatic fringe consists of sixty-eight per cent of the people!' This teacher, who lectured for several days a week and ran a substantial private practice, was at home in the school and out of sympathy with his professional colleagues. He spoke of attending a meeting of practitioners in his area:

> They are a religious lot, in the main, and I realised that I have nothing in common with them. They are only interested in the weird, the exotic and the wonderful. The usual sort of chiropractic meeting reminds me of an Amway seminar. My interest in marketing lies in another direction. I should run courses for doctors on spinal manipulation. That would be a good thing to do, to teach them what it's about and how to do it.

Staff who were disaffected with school management favoured the unfettered admission of guest speakers. They saw themselves as outsiders (speaking critically of 'the administration', 'it' and 'them' as they conveyed their distance from school leaders). Even when they had as little sympathy as other teachers for sectoral preoccupations and systems, they did not deny the profession. One had fallen out with SOT and other 'unscientific' practitioners in earlier years, leading to a vigorous correspondence with them in the local newsletter. In the course of it, a practitioner argued that while the teacher questioned the scientific basis of the chiropractic nerve interference concept, he could be answered within the framework of 'new' science:

> Quantum Mechanics is now turning upside down many of our long held mechanistic Newtonian views of our world and what is in it, or thought to be in it . . .

> Mechanistic evaluation is becoming the dinosaur of science. Vitalism is slowly being accepted within the scientific community as an integral part of the evaluative procedures — difficult as it may be for left brain dominant people to accept — again I am not judging or labelling anyone, as it is all in the eye of the beholder. . . .

> I am greatly concerned at what appears to be a reversal within our profession because of left brain mechanistic thinking . . .

The left brain (male — analytical side) is what has got our world into such a mess — What is needed is quality right brain (feminine — intuitive, creative) people to become our new leaders.

Our profession should be in the forefront of the new science, not following in the footsteps of an outmoded mechanistic medical model which has taken the feeling out of healing.[20]

The teacher responded by editorialising that vitalism could not be linked with holism, new science and quantum physics: chiropractic had begun with a vitalistic theory but had 'then watered this down to holistic and homeostatic concepts as the science of chiropractic had evolved. It is the opinion of the editor that chiropractic is more appropriately aligned to the theory of holism and NOT VITALISM'.[21] But this dispute had its influence. The teacher explained:

The profession has difficulty with me because I'm a maverick within [chiropractic] orthodoxy. One of the outcomes of that exchange of letter-writing is that I'm much more prepared to listen to other views. I trace my current opinions [in support of] having outside speakers in the college back to that.

Only a minority of students had sympathy for, or espoused, the ideas promoted by straights, SOT practitioners, and others deemed unscientific or excessively philosophical by the school. But many felt they were missing out on chiropractic. They disliked school control. The widespread opinion was that the school ruled their lives. Forty (of the fifty-five) second-year students told the school executive committee they had some negative feelings towards the course and that a lack of enthusiasm was prevalent. The emphasis seemed to be on what chiropractic could not do rather than on what it could do:

This combined with other factors seems to have led to a negative, almost 'anti-Chiropractic' feeling within the class. We feel we need to try and understand the potential of Chiropractic and believe it totally reasonable to expect that Chiropractic be presented in a much more positive light.

Many people feel the 'philosophy' aspect of the course has been portrayed in a negative way, to the extent of almost 'knocking' the founders. While we know that adjusting the subluxation alone can't cure everything, the reasons for adjusting and the results it does achieve should be well highlighted. It is this which has led Chiropractic to be the 'separate and distinct' profession it is. We also recognise that while the founders may have been wrong at times, they must have contributed in many ways to the growth and survival of Chiropractic.[22]

The students sought guest lectures by field practitioners about their 'grassroots' experiences, and by prominent professional identities on current local and overseas issues. They also wanted non-examinable lectures on the basic chiropractic philosophies 'which still apply today and [are] still respected as a cornerstone of our profession and serves as an important part in our understanding of Chiropractic today'. Molloy's moment was arriving.

The executive referred the submission to the chiropractic sciences department.[23] It chided students for poor attendance at guest lectures and advised them that 'prominent professionals' would be included in 1989, as had been the case in 1988.[24] That avoided the issue. The students wanted to hear from the chiropractors that the school kept out, not the ones it let in. The complaints were hardly new. Students had made similar proposals eight years before. They asked for the inclusion of more philosophic principles from the works of the founders of chiropractic and greater contact with field practitioners 'perhaps by inviting Chiropractors onto campus as guest lecturers'.[25] Some had been admitted then but the subsequent hardening of the 'line' indicated a consolidation of authority in the school and leadership estimations of the threat posed to rational chiropractic by the likes of Molloy. In turn, that gave rise to a principle which drew students and sympathetic staff together: their catch-cry was 'freedom of speech'.

One staff interpretation was that students had perennial concerns which existed more or less independently of any earlier action to remedy deficiencies:

> Whenever the students complain and you ask them what specifically is wrong with it, the only answer you sort of get is about getting outside lecturers in, about having a positive view of it, not that there is anything really in the stuff that they get that is wrong that they can pinpoint. And there is a change with the practitioners that they don't realise — they go out there and practise and need to be enthused about what they are doing, to feel it is important and worthwhile. And that's what they get from these seminars, from people like Dr. Parker [another famous American chiropractic evangelist whose approach was not favoured in the school], who might not actually say much when you analyse it, but who make the people feel good about what they are doing. I'm all for having the practitioners here to do that.

Other staff thought that students had unreal expectations or misplaced prior conceptions about chiropractic and they were obliged to face up to them in the course: 'They are looking to a simplified theory they can accept. A lot of them come in here with some idea of what it is all about. They think they know, and that can be a problem.'

Again, there was the staff idea that students did not understand their academic purpose. As one of the lecturers put it, the job of teachers in institutions of higher education was to present an across-the-range view and to test and question the various positions. It was the same with chiropractic techniques, he said. Students went to a seminar, saw enthusiasm for a new technique and came back:

> all fired up to do it and wanting to know why we don't. And we are saying, 'well, it hasn't been validated yet; there is no work done so far about its efficacy and success'. And the students get upset that we are not positive.

The open-debate argument won out and a guest lecturer programme was arranged for the next year (1989). Even Molloy was allowed but only after hard dispute at a chiropractic sciences staff meeting and nearly over the dean's dead body. A teacher told me that when the possibility of having Molloy was raised: '[The dean] said we had to be careful who we let into the school and [a colleague] and I jumped on him about freedom of speech'. The speakers still had to be listed in advance and approved by the school, and the programme had to be 'balanced' (that is, contain acceptable as well as unacceptable practitioners). A further condition was that (as another teacher put it) 'staff attended so they could counter bullshit'. The speakers were not allowed into classes. Instead, they occupied a 'common free time' hour once a week at mid-day.

The 'correct procedure' for inviting outside speakers on the campus was still being disputed at the start of the following year (1990).[26] Another school graduate, who was supposed to have got into trouble with the registration board for allowing a student to practise without supervision during a field placement, had been set down to give a talk and the dean was strongly opposed. His argument was that the executive committee had responsibility for school management and therefore it should decide who was to be invited to speak 'on behalf of the Institute' (the old argument that the school had a duty to act *in loco parentis* — a contention that was not backed by any warrant to exclude speakers on Phillip's behalf).

The debate had started in the diagnostic sciences department, where the 'free-speechers' had the numbers, but the dean had moved it out, arguing, so a teacher said, 'that it was a confidential matter that had to be settled by the executive committee'. As often happened with contentious issues, the executive never got around to the matter. It was delayed or put aside because there was insufficient time. When a staff member did press for consideration by the executive, the two sides were put but the discussion was inconclusive. The day afterwards, a teacher told me:

> The school has this tendency to excommunicate people it doesn't like — to cut them off from everything. The only way to handle [the dean] is to appeal to a principle he can't get around, in this case, the principle of free speech. That's something I've learned. I intend to tell the students this programme is under threat. Why should I be stirring the students up? There's the way in which a radical organisation, one on the margins of science, so far as science is concerned, itself becomes ultra-conservative. That's something that is bad for chiropractic — protecting itself against any freedom of action.

As the executive had noted in passing, the students themselves might invite speakers. This they proceeded to do. In response to what they saw as oppressive school control over the guest programme the students cut out the school and ran the Wednesday lectures themselves. Having once allowed the possibility of a broader programme, continuing school attempts to regulate the series were all too obvious. Both the staff who were prepared to give the philosophers and systems proponents a hearing and the students who resented being 'protected' found school concessions insufficient.

Soon after the chiropractic students' association took over the guest lecturer programme, its president was complaining that the issue of common free time 'had raised its ugly head again'.[27] There was no longer an hour of the week when students were free to get together for guest lectures and other events:

> The CSA [Chiropractic Students' Association] is a group of students, committed to Chiropractic and trying to make the School a better place, who are now starting to ask why are we bothering???? when yet another force acting against us appears to be the Administration. As a student body it's maybe about time we took some affirmative action.

Molloy continued to seek (and to be denied) the access he took to be his due. He proferred his services as a supervisor for field placements but received no school answer. The staff member who arranged these placements said that if he was asked by students about working with Molloy, he told them that they might seek to do so but predicted that any application would be refused (which meant that no student did apply). This teacher told me he believed every registered practitioner should be eligible to take students unless they had demonstrated their unsuitability, which Molloy had not. Was Molloy banned then? 'Well, yes', said the teacher, 'there's no way [the dean] will have him'. A shared understanding of external antagonism and embattlement created an astute, tough leadership and provided the justification for it. Molloy appreciated that as well or better than most. I said to him that the dean had not *formally* banned him. 'No', Molloy replied, 'but remember, you are dealing with one of the smartest people around'.

FREE SPEECH

The dean gave a free-time student talk a week before Molloy made his first appearance in the series. No less than Molloy and Gold, he set out to generate enthusiasm for chiropractic. Students were urged to have 'faith, confidence and belief in your products, services and ideas'. That was borrowed from Dr. Parker, the dean said. He used the saying to convey his main point: students would be limiting their products, services and ideas if they stuck to one technique system. If they did use procedures that were not part of the mainstream, certain elements of SOT or AK, for example, they should be cautious, as doctors were with a new procedure or a new drug. They should never make it the centre of their practice: 'Remember the basic mosaic of the stuff that's proven, the things that we know to work'. The dean turned to the Innate:

> On the issue of faith, some of you were referred here to the course by practitioners who say if you don't follow Innate Intelligence you won't get the Big Idea. The question of faith becomes all important in relation to the amount of knowledge . . . Let us see whether when you leave here you can depend more on our knowledge than on faith. Twenty to thirty years ago, you had to have faith because you identified a subluxation and adjusted and it worked but now we know more. Let us include *knowledge* in this little formula for an additional approach to what we do in private practice.

They needed persistence. The dean remembered:

Thirty years ago at a Palmer college homecoming there was a chiropractor who was so burdened down he was ready to chuck it in. He rang up B.J. expecting support but he said — 'When you get to the end of the rope, tie a knot and hang on' — and hung up. It's a story about deficits: this professional person lacked one quality; it was persistence.

Molloy's speech was something of an anti-climax. The prodigal son was as enthusiastic as the dean but he steered well clear of straights philosophy. There was a *mea culpa* for his own lack of learning as a student, which had obliged him to spend 'hundreds of thousands of dollars' to make up later. He urged the students to work hard at college. They had to know where they were going and what they were doing:

Jim Parker talks about having faith, confidence and belief in your products, services and ideas. What is needed is responsibility, commitment and determination. B.J. Palmer had a saying — 'You never know how far reaching what you say, do and think today will affect the lives of millions tomorrow' — that includes what you don't say, do or think today.

Molloy wanted to know how his lecture had been received when I saw him later in one of the student clinics (he was 'visiting'). I said there was little to choose between him and the dean when it came to inspirational messages but he had not delivered a Sherman college style of talk, as many students expected. Molloy could trim his sails to fit the wind. He said: 'Having got in, I was not about to risk staying in by doing any such thing!' The dean was alert to that. He wanted to know about Molloy's talk. When I told him Molloy had not mentioned 'straights' philosophy, the dean replied: 'He's just doing that, I bet, so he can get a foot in the door!' The next year, Molloy was back again for a lunch-time seminar (entitled 'What Makes Us Special'). This time, the students asked him in.

CONCLUSION

Chiropractors were fearful about their future. They nearly all agreed that 'political' medicine was set on destroying their occupation. Reggie had asked: 'How the hell do you build a profession in the face of such opposition? If you were the only chiropractor left on earth, would chiropractic survive?' His answer, and Molloy's, was to make no concessions and to affirm the rebellious distinctiveness of chiropractic. They invoked its pristine ethicality: people who had been touched by the Big Idea could renew their allegiance, however much they had tainted it and had themselves been tainted by admixture. Here was optimism in perfectability, and a heady message for students. They could be confident in themselves because they *were* chiropractors. It was tough but the black chiropractor had it tougher. Their minority status was their strength.

The other answer, which the school had adopted, involved raising the occupation up in a different way: medicine would come to accept chiropractic when it realised how well equipped the graduates were to take their place alongside other health care practitioners. That required a different sort of faith. Would the denigration of chiropractic ever cease? Adrift in such a perilous sea, many students and graduates clung onto any rope of certitude they could find.

In aligning with philosophical thinking, students also rebelled against the dominations of the school. It was scarcely a case of repudiating science but of putting it in its place. Few graduates might become committed straights — Molloy told me the CSA membership stood at 'about thirteen' (out of the two thousand registered Australian chiropractors) — but many would end up with an animus to the school which its shielding of them had helped to instil.

Notes

(Unless otherwise noted, documents are from School of Chiropractic and Osteopathy archives and working files).
1. Molloy, T. to Drinkwater, J. (ACCE executive secretary), 10 July 1986.
2. Molloy, T. to Kleynhans, A., 11 April 1986.
3. 'Constitution of the Chiropractic Society of Australia'. n.d., pp. 1-2.
4. School of Chiropractic. 'Institutional Self-Evaluation Update', September 1984.
5. File note by Campbell, S. (then school registrar), 29.April 1985.
6. Molloy, T. to Drinkwater, J., 10 July 1986.
7. 'Renaissance, A New Age Seminar'. n.d. (c.1979).
8. Minutes, Executive Committee, 19 March 1985.
9. Minutes, Executive Committee, 25 March 1985.
10. Minutes, Chiropractic Sciences Department, 24 April 1985.
11. Kleynhans, A. Memo to staff, 26 April 1985.
12. Molloy, T. to Drinkwater, J., 10 July 1986
13. Minutes, Executive Committee, 5 November 1985.
14. Minutes, Executive Committee, 28 January 1986.
15. Kleynhans, A. to Molloy, T., 10 December 1976. Molloy's records.
16. Charlton, K. 'Chiropractic and the Gold Standard'. *A.C.A. Newsletter* 6, 1, 9 (1986). The title is a play on Bloch's calling randomised controlled trials the 'gold standard of experimental design' (1987, 430). Bloch reviewed the methodologies used in clinical back pain studies and concluded that only a few

met this standard.

17. 'Acetabular Proprioceptors', attachment to *Chairman's Corner – The Newslettter of the Sacro-Occipital Technique Organisation (A/Sia.) Ltd.*, August 1989, pp. 1-4.

18. Ames, R. Letter to the Editor *A.C.A. News* 16, 8 (October/November 1989), 4-5.

19. In SOTO brochure 'Winter Research Symposium July 3, 4 and 5 [1989]', referring to a presentation by Leyonhjelm, K., the SOTO Chairman. He also mentioned 'a 30 second adjustment to eliminate Candida' in the December 1988 edition of *Chairman's Corner*, p. 2. Subsequently, Leyonhjelm responded to a critic who spoke ironically of chiropractic alchemy: he would have been prepared to accept a criticism for adjusting symptoms but not one 'for a chiropractor believing that an "adjustment" could possibly help a patient eliminate from his being an affliction/disease that previously had been only ever controlled by the ingestion of some form of "medicine"'. April 1989 edition of *Chairman's Corner*, pp. 1-2.

20. Powell, A. Letter to the Editor, *ACA Victorian Branch News Bulletin*, 8, 5 (May 1987), 16-17.

21. Editorial, *ACA Victorian Branch News Bulletin*, 8, 5 (May 1987), 3.

22. 'Statement from the Year Two Chiropractic Class', 2 September 1988.

23. Minutes, Executive Committee, 20 September 1988.

24. Minutes, Chiropractic Sciences Staff Meeting, 27 October 1988.

25. 'International College of Chiropractic Students Association, Course Evaluation Sub-Committee, Interim Report on: Structure and Organisation of the PIT/ICC B.App.Sci. (Chiropractic) Degree', 27 November 1980

26. Minutes, Executive Committee, 15 March 1990.

27. 'From the President's Pen', *The Axis*, vol. 5, 23 July 1990.

V

BATTLING THE ESTABLISHMENT

Medical care in Australia is based on concepts of 'disease' — its diagnosis, treatment and prevention. Within this framework of medical care acupuncture DOES NOT provide a means of DIAGNOSIS or prevention of disease.

(Draft Consumer Information Brochure in *Report*, National Health and Medical Research Council Working Party on Acupuncture in Westerman, 1988, 1989, vii.)

INTRODUCTION

The NH&MRC, a federal statutory body, looms large in the financing of medical research in the universities and research institutes. Also, it issues statements on health, safety and standards. Usually these are commissioned by standing committees and prepared by expert groups, with members drawn from universities and the medical profession and supported by medical staff in the Commonwealth Department of Community Services and Health (DCSH). The council itself only meets several times a year.

An NH&MRC working party was appointed to scrutinise acupuncture in 1987. Its report (Westerman, 1988) and a later revision (1989) came out strongly against 'non-medical' or 'lay' practitioners.[1] This chapter deals with the fight to overturn the working party reports. Though the NH&MRC had no formal say about registration and the commencement of higher education courses, interlocking governmental, professional and academic representation made its advice influential. The NH&MRC could not dispose of traditional acupuncture but it was in a position to abet or check the causes of its advocates.

SCIENCE, SAFETY, DANGER

There was much in the reports to confirm traditional acupuncturists in the belief that the working party had set out to damage them. Doctors practising acupuncture were exempted from criticism and commended for their offer of proper diagnosis and safe treatment. This was particularly galling, since the traditional acupuncturists knew how few had more than a brief instructional acquaintance with acupuncture technique, and even less education in traditional theory.

A death following treatment by an unregistered acupuncture practitioner ten years previously had been the subject of a coronial inquiry. The working party used it to substantiate the dangers of acupuncture in other than medical hands. As the traditional acupuncturists discovered, the working party's citation for its account, a newspaper article about the coronial proceedings, did not bear out its contention. The working party gave the impression that the acupuncturist had caused the death by penetrating both lungs with long needles. The newspaper reported the coroner as saying he did not believe this was likely. On the testimony of the forensic pathologist, he found the cause of death to be emphysema and a myocardial infarction. Traditional practitioners associated with the Australian Acupuncture College in Melbourne (who, at any rate, had nothing to do with the practitioner involved in the coronial inquiry) maintained they were judged by association and on the misrepresentation of one case.

Having obtained access to the federal health department's acupuncture working party papers under the Freedom of Information Act, I found that many of the complaints by traditional acupuncturists were justified (see O'Neill, 1990, 1991a, for detailed reviews). The association representing medical practitioners of acupuncture, the Australian Medical Acupuncture Society (AMAS) had privileged access to the working party, including a nominated member. It wanted governments to ban the practice of 'lay' acupuncture. Many assertions about traditional acupuncturists in the working party's correspondence, and in background papers prepared by the secretariat, lacked evidentiary foundation. While submissions were invited and obtained from traditional acupuncture organisations, the working party did not inspect private colleges and relied on damaging generalisations about their staff, students and courses by medical practitioners who had not visited them either.

Before its first report the working party had not even seen the cited newspaper account of the coronial inquiry. This version said:

> In 1970, it was alleged in the Coroner's Court in Melbourne that a lay acupuncturist had used a very long needle at this point on one side, resulting in the collapse of the patient. The acupuncturist used a needle of the same length on the other side to attempt to revive the patient. The patient died because both lung cavities had been pierced, causing both lungs to collapse (Bilateral pneumothoraces). (*The Age* 1970)'.[2]

The NH&MRC's health care committee sent the report back to the working party for further consideration but not in relation to this allegation. In between-times, and after a search by the secretariat, a ten years-on newspaper article about the case was discovered. The second published version (Westerman, 1988, 60) retained the words of the first, with the newspaper citation changed to 'Lynch, 1980' — referring to an article by this reporter in another newspaper, *The Australian*, on 2 September 1980. No-one seems to have checked that the newly discovered source actually said what the text averred. As several working party members told me, they all knew about the case. Word about it (rather, selected convictions about 'the facts') had passed around: here, as with chiropractors, a general view about the danger of non-medical operatives was readily confirmed. I concluded that the working party had relied on word-of-mouth reports for their mistaken account.

Even after the acupuncturists had demonstrated the errors and a transcript of the proceedings had been obtained for the working party, the final report of the working party (Westerman, 1989, 71) continued to be inaccurate about the case. The working party still used the Lynch article as a citation for a report in the press that the patient died after both lungs had been pierced by acupuncture needles. Then the following appeared: 'However, for various technical reasons the forensic pathologist was unable to confirm or refute whether the cause of death was directly related to acupuncture, but it was clear from the transcript of the case and from the Coroner's findings that prior to treatment the patient was seriously ill' (Westerman, 1989, 71). The transcript does not bear out this interpretation. The pathologist's evidence about the cause of death was clear. As to needle marks, he said he had seen none nor would expect to have done so: it was hard enough to find hypodermic needle marks, much less those of acupuncture needles.

Did this mean the working party was out to 'get' the traditional acupuncturists? My view, that members were not so much maliciously inclined as misled by blunt certitudes about *their* science, nearly brought relations with the principal of the Melbourne college to an end. To suggest that the reports displayed a convenient ineptitude but not necessarily a destructive intent was to side with the working party. The principal responded angrily. He said the first published report (the second was yet to be issued) was a tissue of fabrications, misleading statements and deceptions: 'They call themselves scientists and what they have done is make up things, lied, deliberately lied. They have set out to destroy acupuncture'. My interpretation was too generous. He said: 'How many people do I have to *kill* to prove it is unsafe?'

That was a crucial point. On the one hand, traditional acupuncturists held that needling at the right places and at the right angles and depths, in the right combination of points and at the right times, did a power of good. The proof was the harm that could result from getting the thing wrong. A college teacher said about the death investigated by the coroner: 'The trouble is, [the practitioner] left the needles in so long she exhausted the poor woman's Qi'. On the other hand, the working party translated a widely publicised risk, of transmitting fatal conditions like AIDS and Hepatitis B with infected needles, into the infective possibilities of consulting lay acupuncturists. (All the traditional acupuncturists I observed used disposable needles. No doubt some were less aseptically rigorous than others but that generalisation applies to practitioners of all sorts. The working party presented an unbalanced account by concentrating on one side: what was or might be the danger of 'lay' acupuncture. There is no evidence that members tried to find out what safety procedures were employed by traditional acupuncturists). The traditional acupuncturists allied the danger of acupuncture with its potency, the working party with the ignorance of its unregistered practitioners.

Still, the working party had a problem. Governments could no longer be relied on to implement proposals to confine the 'non-medical' practice of acupuncture;[3] and the working party itself was not about to confer legitimacy on lay acupuncturists by proposing that they be registered and educated in universities. The working party believed that: 'The safest option for the community would be to restrict the practice of acupuncture to medical practitioners' (1989, 71). But it said that recommending a ban on lay acupuncture would no longer be acceptable, being seen as a relic of medical paternalism.

Having discarded that, the working party said: 'the community is now faced with the principle of Caveat Emptor (let the buyer beware) in making health decisions and treatment choices' (1989, 76).

This shifted the problem onto consumers, which was rather undermined by the working party's harking on dangers, such as the 'more subtle risk' of acupuncture analgesia masking symptoms and so delaying the diagnosis of conditions like spine and brain tumours (1979, 70). The case for registration and higher education had to be proportionate to the risks, subtle and otherwise: that was no more than the obverse of the proposition that doctors were best because their scientific training enabled them to deliver safe acupuncture. Therefore the more dangerous acupuncture could be shown to be, the more evident it would also be that governments had to take action 'in the interests of public safety'.

EDUCATION

The traditional acupuncture colleges in Melbourne and Sydney advanced what they held to be an uncorrupted form of traditional Chinese medicine. Leaders said that even in China it had been compromised by western medical additions. Everything in this medicine might have its basis in the classics but recognition could not be obtained without the inclusion of western medical sciences taught, if possible, by 'reputable' higher education institutions.

Having decided to seek state government accreditation for its course, the Sydney college gained assistance from an advanced education institution which, for money, presented western medical sciences courses to students. This connection paid off and the course was certified. Following that example, the Melbourne college approached the Lincoln Institute of Health Sciences and settled a contract for the teaching of western medical science subjects. An arrangement had been in place for several years before the NH&MRC got interested in acupuncture again.

The Sydney and Melbourne principals agreed that students hated western medical sciences. The former said: 'We will do as little western medical science as we can get away with — no more than a third of the course, in fact it's a quarter.' The Melbourne principal explained the compromise to students:

In the same way that traditional Chinese diagnosis is not relevant for the practice of western medicine, so western diagnosis is not relevant for the practice of TCM. We include it [in the course] to exclude conditions that should be treated by other health practitioners; to make you aware of things we are not allowed to treat; and because all health practitioners should be health practitioners first and specialists second. Western medical sciences is needed for any practitioner in the western world today.

As the Melbourne principal told an earlier group of students:

We thought that government authorities and the medical profession as a whole would hold it against us unless institutions, rather than individuals, however good [at TCM], did western medical sciences. In a sense, by doing that we were able to assure health authorities we were at least safe. Further, it helped us get an accredited programme [i.e. that offered by the Sydney college].

In collaboration with some teachers in the Lincoln Institute biological sciences department (who presented the western medical sciences courses), the Melbourne acupuncture college then developed an undergraduate acupuncture degree proposal. Lincoln was in the midst of merger negotiations with La Trobe and the idea was that the acupuncture course would travel into the university with the Institute. At first, the aim had been to secure registration and a higher education berth so that traditional acupuncture could flourish in its pristine form. Now leaders sought a partnership for acupuncturists in the old firm. The principal told new students in 1989 that registration was just around the corner. He said it was important for safety reasons because the profession would be protected, and:

The other important thing is the incorporation of the course into La Trobe. That will ensure standards, open the opportunities for funded research programmes, Masters and Ph Ds, and that will only enhance our entry to the Australian health care system. It will bring acupuncture into the respectable area of education and so also into the Australian health care system.

Lincoln physiotherapists opposed the course, using the same formula they advanced against chiropractic years before. They maintained that the body of knowledge was insufficient to occupy a full degree, and that 'The judgment in respect to the body of knowledge and/or skills required should remain in the hands of the experts — i.e. medical and health practitioners and scientists — and not the general public, government or administrators'. They went on to say that medical practitioners, veterinary scientists, physiotherapists and dentists already had the knowledge required to apply acupuncture safely and appropriately, and that 'a post-graduate diploma would be sufficient to learn the *practice* of acupuncture'.[4] Offering acupuncture was even a moral imperative. Arguing that the Australian Physiotherapy Association (APA) should place no barrier in the way of members practising acupuncture, Dix (1985, 208) said: 'There are other practitioners, of all shades, holding themselves out as acupuncturists and patients must not be forced to seek them out'.

Following the 1988 transfer of Lincoln to La Trobe University, the university would decide on the introduction of an undergraduate acupuncture course. Six months after the issue of the first NH&MRC report, the course proposal went to La Trobe's academic board. It foundered, despite endorsement by the senior university staff who had attended the college graduation a little while before. The NH&MRC report was cited as evidencing scientific unworthiness. The dean of one of the science schools suggested that a postgraduate course for medical practitioners might be an acceptable alternative. He doubted there was enough in acupuncture to warrant a full undergraduate degree. Besides, if acupuncture were to be allowed, 'it opens the doors to things like hypnosis coming into the university'. As soon as a Lincoln behavioural scientist member stated that acupuncture had not been scientifically validated and that the research papers she had seen were methodologically unsound, the other members backed off. Apart from the Lincoln dean, none of them spoke in favour of the course and some members from the La Trobe science schools spoke against it.

When he heard the proposal had been withdrawn for want of support, a Lincoln teacher who had helped develop the course said about the scientists who had opposed its introduction: 'Bunch of pricks, they shouldn't be allowed to wear clothes! They should have to sit there with nothing on while they make their lofty speeches!' That was how the traditional acupuncturists felt about it too. They as frequently ran into academic as into medical opposition. The director of an interstate alternative medicines college put it this way: 'Because we are on the fringe of medicine and on the fringe of education we have powerful forces opposed to us in both camps. It's a sort of double whammy!'

Ingrained convictions of the truth-equals-science kind were foremost whenever registration or the institution of higher education courses were blocked. A Victorian parliamentary committee (Dixon,

1986, vol.1, 181) said that registering the alternatives would imply
government endorsement of a body of knowledge that had not been
established by scientific inquiry and therefore it could not
'recommend *de facto* recognition of these therapies by registration of
practitioners'. The AMA submission to this committee had been
forthright:

> All forms of unscientific medicine should be discouraged and the
> very worst thing that could happen with respect to alternative
> medicine is that it be given any form of official recognition by the
> Government (in Dixon, 1986, vol.1, 175).

The committee also endorsed a recommendation about the
registration of health professionals made at a 1981 conference of the
Australian state and federal health ministers:

> a health services provider group should be registered where there is
> a potential to cause serious physical harm, or death, to a recipient
> of the services or in respect of which significant Government
> payments are made (in Dixon, 1986, vol.1, 178).

The working party's assertions about acupuncture not being
scientifically validated counted with the academics for not proceeding
with a course in it but the extensive comments about lay acupuncture
dangers might count with the politicians for regulating it. As the
principal of the Australian Acupuncture College in Melbourne told
me: 'When we are making submisssions about registration we can
come in with the NH&MRC report tucked under our arms, saying "it
is harmful!"'.

MOBILISING OPPOSITION

Compared to the divisions between chiropractors when they were
fighting for recognition, the traditional acupuncturists were in even
greater organisational disarray. There were other gloomy signs.
Colleges struggled to get enough students. Leading figures in some
of them were opposed to regulation. If the Sydney and Melbourne
Australian Acupuncture College camp obtained higher education
courses and seats on registration boards then they were expected to
cut the ground from under internal competitors. The proprietor of a
college in another state said:

The drop-kick in the testicles will come in the form of registration and that will come in the form of requiring standards. That will drive out of business a lot of places and opportunities for study and a place like yours [La Trobe University] will take over. The reason they are getting rid of their colleges [i.e. seeking to transfer courses to higher education] is that they can't run them. They can't get the money together to get adequate staff and facilities. They can't generate the funds to run a proper college and they want to get the monkey off their back. They hope they will be offered wonderful jobs in universities. It's the old principle: you capitalise the profit industries and you socialise the loss industries . . . I'm the lone voice against registration: would you trust doctors from the health department and lawyers from crown law to make laws for us? They will standardise us out of business. The moment you regulate an occupation you close it off, same as chiropractic. It doesn't help the consumer.

Many traditional acupuncture interest groups made submissions to the working party but after its first published report only two groups — a combination of the Acupuncture Ethics and Standards Organisation (AESO) and the Sydney and Melbourne colleges, and the Australian Natural Therapists Association (ANTA) — presented substantial responses. The ANTA submission argued that the working party had dealt with education and training:

so superficially, peremptorily and one-sidedly, that it could only lead to one apparently preconceived conclusion, namely the neutralisation and thereby the eventual elimination of non-medical acupuncturists by stating that 'The safest option for the community would be to restrict the practice of acupuncture to medical practitioners'.[5]

While the college acupuncturists agreed with ANTA about the report, they were at daggers drawn over everything else and did not get together to fight the NH&MRC.[6] The whole conduct of the battle lay with an AESO/college lobby group called the 'Committee for the Evaluation of the N. H. & M. R. C.'s Report on Acupuncture'. The principals of the Sydney and Melbourne colleges were the fiery particles of its existence, circulating all the expressions of shock and dismay. A few other dedicated acupuncturists, never more than four, helped them by cataloguing the failings, combing the research literature and producing extensive commentaries. What the committee lacked in numbers and influence, it made up for in the volume and insistence of its utterances.

For all their conviction and unquenchable public optimism, the college principals sometimes despaired privately. Running the fight was extremely demanding. It was not so much the medical enemy but the failure of your own people to live up to expectations that was corrosive. The course proposal was about to go to the La Trobe University academic board and, the Melbourne College principal said, the profession was unconcerned. He had just been to a meeting of the Australian Traditional Medicine Society (ATMS), a broad association whose membership was not confined to traditional Chinese practitioners. The colleges had pulled out of it:

> We are in conflict with others over our different philosophy. But so far as [the ATMS] is concerned, it's almost better not to have us in there. Basically, they don't want regulation or government involvement. They are a bunch of small businessmen who share small business views about government intervention. They really sit around debating whether naturopathy and natural therapies are different, and whether or not naturopathy exists.

The danger with the Australian Natural Therapists Association (ANTA), the other big group with a general cover, was its putting acupuncture in with other therapies. The principal ruled out any association:

> If acupuncture merged with naturopathy it would lose its depth and become a cook-book style therapy. Acupuncture and traditional Chinese medicine would lose its unique place and would be restricted to a technique. It would lose its heart, its system.

Leaders spoke of the absorptive aims of ANTA — which had an accreditation board with a traditional Chinese medicine sub-committee — in much the same terms as they spoke of the equivalent intentions of established medicine.[7]

The situation within AESO was hardly better. AESO was an accrediting body but it was the nearest thing these traditional acupuncturists had to a professional association. As such the leaders thought it was a failure. The members just did not care. The principal said about AESO:

> It's always been a dictator; a *benevolent* dictator. They [traditional acupuncturists] are as apathetic as hell: most people are only interested in themselves. We have very self-interested practitioners unfortunately . . . AESO has been trying to run the AESO society of practitioners, hoping the profession would learn to establish a

professional association. Getting the bloody profession to turn up to anything they do is bloody difficult.

In addition, the principal said, college teachers were already jockeying for future positions at La Trobe University. After cataloguing external antagonists, internal difficulties and turmoils, the principal exclaimed: 'Is it worth struggling on? Often my mind screams — let it go'.

The unconcern of all but a few within meant that decisions had to be taken unilaterally. The Sydney principal said of AESO:

> Perhaps it's not democratic, some say that, but where there are democratic organisations, as in Queensland, they do nothing for acupuncture.[8] They spend their energy on seeking votes and maintaining voting blocs for election. I cannot understand the apathy of AESO members. They expect everything to be done for them by AESO. When we had the votes for the AESO practitioners association there were seven positions and only five votes overall. Some did not even vote for themselves! AESO is a dictatorship, in one sense, because it does all the work. But other people in the profession are not prepared to do it. They ring up and complain when there is something critical about acupuncture in the newspaper, but you never get one call when you have achieved something.

The principals felt they carried the largely unrespected and unsupported burden of action. Only they could get things done when the membership lacked any corporate concern, was lazy and selfish. But it was not possible for members (those who had been accredited and paid the annual fee) to become engaged in the conduct of AESO and no doubt their passivity was related to their lack of influence over its affairs.[9]

AESO was started as a means of certifying practitioners so their patients could obtain reimbursement from private health insurance funds.[10] This, and the arrangement of practitioner indemnity insurance, continued to be the membership advantages. A loyalty condition was introduced some six years later. One of the ANTA leaders (himself a graduate of the Sydney college) had courtesy accreditation with AESO from its inception. In 1983 he was advised that a new clause had been inserted in the AESO code of ethics and he would be expected to observe it.[11] The clause began:

In the interest of unity within the acupuncture profession, no accreditee may publicly denigrate the AESO, its Board of Chairmen and Governors, its Accrediting Committee, office bearers or appointees.[12]

The penalty for non-observance was the withdrawal of accreditation status. Nearly always, 'in the interests of unity' statements indicated the existence of considerable disunity, prefaced measures that were liable to continue it, and imposed limitations intended to tighten the membership boundary.

AESO also elevated its entry requirements. After the Sydney college gained course accreditation, the provisions were altered so that : (i) automatic recognition was restricted to graduates of Australian government accredited courses or overseas courses deemed equivalent; (ii) students in other Australian colleges could only sit for AESO admission examinations if (a) their colleges were undergoing the process of government accreditation, (b) all their western medical sciences components were taught by government-accredited universities or colleges of advanced education, and (c) the colleges submitted course details to AESO and it was satisfied they were similar in length and content to the Sydney college course.[13]

Overseas candidates apart, the effect of these changes was to limit membership eligibility to the graduates of the Sydney and Melbourne colleges since no others met conditions (ii) (a) and (b); and (ii) (c), at any rate, demanded a surrender to AESO. In Parkin's terms (1974; 1979) moves to restrict membership amounted to the adoption of an exclusionary closure strategy: benefits accruing from the professionalisation of acupuncture would be reserved for members and those who were not in the AESO camp would be shut out. But this does not capture the meaning of the restrictions for those who were intent on introducing them. Leaders were convinced that acupuncture had to be lifted to reputability by demonstrating that some practitioners did have standards, and they were determined to make every post a winning post. The chase took on its own momentum.

Each gain was made into a springboard for another. After the Sydney college got a tertiary institution to offer western medical sciences, the Melbourne college cited the arrangement as a precedent when it asked Lincoln Institute to do the same. New South Wales accreditation was used to advance the case for transferring the Sydney college course to the tertiary institution that offered western medical sciences to acupuncture students. When negotiations looked to be going well in Sydney, Lincoln was invited to follow suit. All previous gains and the elevation of AESO qualification requirements (which had been based on them) were then used to evidence registration suitability.

To complete the circle, approaches from other groups representing acupuncturists or offering acupuncture courses were denied. Saying that it was holding out the hand of friendship on behalf of the whole profession and patients for much needed mutual professional co-operation, ANTA invited AESO to nominate members to its accreditation board.[14] AESO would have none of it. A nearby college of natural therapies and traditional Chinese medicine suggested a meeting with the Sydney college 'to discuss possible areas of co-operation and collaboration and the potential for friendly relations'.[15] The college advised that it was in the midst of arranging the transfer of its acupuncture programme to a university and that 'These negotiations . . . have curtailed our freedom to make collaborative arrangements with teaching organisations outside the recognised government tertiary education system in New South Wales'.[16] The Sydney principal said to me: 'When they write and want to be friends, you know they are on the skids'. AESO and the two colleges had made the running and they wanted to keep it that way.

The failure to achieve a national professional association limited the capacity of acupuncturists to mobilise practitioners and patients in campaigns for recognition. And their disunity was used against them. The working party said that course variability indicated:

> a lack of agreement amongst acupuncture organisations as to the nature of the practice of acupuncture and the standards of education required. Clearly, such organisations need to resolve their internal divisions before any uniform accreditation or registration becomes possible (Westerman, 1989, 69).

The Sydney and Melbourne College principals were altogether aware of the problem but they found it hard to understand how they were to be criticised. Why should AESO and their colleges, which had attempted to make a standard, have any truck with sub-standard colleges and organisations? To move towards unity was to put at risk the gains their obduracy had helped to secure. Besides, it was a tactical question and one had to read the mind of the 'real' opponent, established medicine. The Melbourne principal told me that he had no philosophical reason for resisting unification negotiations with other organisations representing traditional acupuncturists, only a political justification. He said:

> Medicine is behind the NH&MRC and it will not give up lightly. It's a matter of recognising that they may be obliged to extend registration but it's a case of where you draw the line or close the door. Of the other [alternative] health occupations, acupuncture is the most 'medicine-like' and so you may extend registration to it but you definitely want to keep the naturopaths and homeopaths out. Therefore any amalgamation move at this stage would definitely be contrary to our project of seeking registration.

The two Victorian chiropractic associations had thought as little of each other and on like grounds, yet they joined together. The difference was that the Sydney and Melbourne principals did not believe the other acupuncture associations and colleges were serious contenders for recognition. Groups forge alliances when unification is specified as a condition of gain or when competition between them is close, the result is uncertain, and the consequence of losing is exclusion from benefits that are near at hand. The principal said AESO and the colleges were being told (by a government senator, see below) that their job was to demonstrate standards, not to amalgamate with others in order to demonstrate unity. 'Mind you', he continued 'if we got the message that we ought to amalgamate to assist registration then we would do that tomorrow. We will do what's necessary, anything at all, but it is not being suggested. We will wait and see.'

The colleges and AESO also established the Australian Council on Acupuncture and Traditional Chinese Medical Education (ACATCME). Like the Australasian Council for Chiropractic Education (ACCE), which provided the model, its purpose was to accredit education programmes and to offer independent education advice to institutions and governments. Traditional acupuncture groups who were opposed to AESO saw ACATCME as no more than another dummy organisation for the college leaders. But it was another piece in the apparatus of respectability, intended to demonstrate to government agencies that AESO practitioners were worthy of licensing and the Sydney and Melbourne colleges worthy of transfer to formal higher education.

There were encouraging signs. Two states appeared to be moving towards the registration of additional groups of health practitioners. The Western Australian health minister said this was his intention a year before the working party made its first report.[17] After an earlier document canvassing the possibilities, his department issued a paper identifying the potential to cause serious harm to the health of a client as the main reason for regulating an occupation.[18] The more recent critical literature on professional monopolies had its influence. The paper said research indicated that legislation restricting practice could reduce consumer choice, raise costs, limit practitioner mobility and restrict job opportunities to certain minorities. It had also been argued that these consequences occurred 'without any necessary concurrent improvement in the quality or safety of regulated activities'. However, omnibus legislation was proposed — with a two-tiered system of title-restricting certification and title and activity-restricting registration. The latter was reserved for occupations demonstrating that they had self-regulating state/national professional associations as opposed to fragmented professional bodies. AESO maintained that it satisfied this condition (the institution of ACATCME providing further evidence) and so ought to qualify for registration rather than certification.[19]

In New South Wales, a discussion paper invited submissions on the statutory regulation of additional health occupations. It also concluded that omnibus registration legislation or the licensing protection of occupational titles were effective means of regulation.[20] Like the West Australian paper, no great emphasis was placed on the science of the occupations. 'I personally feel the future is going to be decided very soon, registration will happen very soon', the principal of the Melbourne college told students. He spoke as if the transfer of the course to La Trobe University would then be a foregone conclusion.

'IT'S ALL GOING TO BE FIXED UP'

The acupuncturists gained assistance from a senator in the federal government party by way of a practitioner who was acquainted with her (she later became interim chairperson of ACATCME). In turn, that led to an interview with the federal health minister, where the 'fabrication' of the coronial report became a central issue.[21] The acupuncturists were bucked-up by this meeting. The message from those attending was that it had been a great victory for acupuncture. The working party had egg on its face; something was going to happen; the minister would roast the working party. The principal speculated about the consequences:

I virtually knew, I felt so strongly when I walked out [of the minister's office] that these people outside were [the members of] the working party . . . This is what I think would have happened after we left the room. [The minister] would have the working party in next. He would say to the chairman — 'You told me that the reference should have been to the coronial inquiry [rather than to the newspaper account] and that the working party report could be adjusted with a word change'. 'Yes' the chairman would have replied. Then the minister would have produced the transcript [of the coronial inquiry, which the acupuncturists had given him] and said — 'Show me'. That would have rocked them; they would have been crawling out under the door. Then he would have raised [the working party's failure to acknowledge that the N.S.W. college course had been accredited by the state government]. That would have broken their backs; he could have got them to do anything. [The minister] said he wanted the NH&MRC membership widened. He would have used this issue to blackmail them. He had them in a corner, I reckon.

The principal expected the working party would now recommend that undergraduate acupuncture courses be introduced in the universities or colleges:

They won't like it any more than they liked doing it for chiropractors but I don't think they will have any choice . . . They can't get rid of us, they have already admitted that. The reality is that we are here to stay.

The working party was a faceless, remote group.[22] Apart from their tenuous contact by way of the senator, the acupuncturists had little to go on. In the twelve months between the issue of the two published versions of the report, they were buoyed by a series of misconceptions about what was being done — supposing others shared the immediacy of their realisation of the worth of acupuncture and of the NH&MRC's unfairness. The expectation was that the minister was going to fix it all up. A letter from the minister to the senator seemed to confirm this.[23] He said the working party had reconvened and had decided to modify its report. Members agreed that registration:

had the potential to distinguish those trained in a 4 year course associated with a tertiary institution from those doing short courses and hence may be of some value in ensuring safe practice of acupuncture. However, as yet, there was no agreed standard which could be applied.

The Working Party supported registration in principle although the conclusions of its report should remain unchanged until there are agreed standards which can be applied.

The minister went on to say that acupuncture organisations had to resolve their internal divisions (over the duration, content and quality of courses) before uniform accreditation became possible, that the working party acknowledged the role in training acupuncturists of the four-year diploma course and was particularly concerned about the safety of those outside AESO, and that deficiencies highlighted in the report 'preclude a recommendation in favour of registration at this stage although the concept is endorsed in principle as a means of ensuring standards and safety'. AESO and the colleges 'should now take action to address these deficiencies as a means of pursuing registration'.

The ire of the acupuncturists was even further aroused when the working party's next report was published six months later. In the main, earlier positions were entrenched by textual modifications. The closest the working party came to making a concession was to lay down heavy qualifications and conditions in the event that governments were 'forced to consider registration of non-medical acupuncturists'. The first of these said:

If legislative bodies are tempted to endorse acupuncture in the interests of medical pluralism, they should do so in the knowledge that as a therapeutic tool acupuncture has been promulgated only on the basis of enthusiasm and anecdotal evidence. As documented in this Report, convincing evidence is lacking of the efficacy of acupuncture per se and free of confounding factors such as observer bias, cultural expectations, patient conviction and placebo effects (Westerman, 1989, 77).

The evaluation committee told the minister that members were 'shocked and dismayed' by the revision and that it was seriously at variance with what he had advised would be the working party's new position.[24] It went on to itemise the working party's continued failure to correctly report the coronial finding; support registration in principle and on safety grounds; recognise that the N.S.W. course had been properly accredited; and mention that ACATCME had been established in order to address the previous concern about the absence of specialist evaluation of diagnostic and biological science course elements.

The minister parried by drawing attention to the continued lack of unity in the profession. He said that the setting up of ACATCME indicated progress but there was still:

fragmentation of organisations claiming to represent acupuncturists and set standards of acupuncture practice . . . The Working Party was not in a position to endorse one group and ignore others, it is for the different acupuncture groups to organise themselves'.[25]

The acupuncturists looked to be back where they started. The working party had dug in over the precondition of occupational unity and over diagnostic incapability (and therefore danger). The latter, especially, raised a hurdle that could not be surmounted without access to the places where students learned the practice of clinical medicine. The minister returned to the distinction in replying to a complaint about the second published report by the dean of the La Trobe Health Sciences School:

A major concern of the working party peparing [sic] this report was to emphasise the need to address, in the development of tertiary courses, those aspects of practice such as clinical diagnosis, microbiology and anatomy, which are essential for safety in the practice of acupuncture. In considering the training of medical practitioners in accupuncture [sic], these issues are not of major concern as they are addressed in the undergraduate medical curiculum [sic].[26]

AESO and the colleges met the professional fragmentation charge with an elaboration of the case presented to the West Australian review. In denying unity in acupuncture training and practitioner accreditation, the working party was said to have ignored AESO's national accreditation standards and its position (along with the two training programmes it recognised) in dealing *exclusively* with acupuncture. The creation of ACATCME demonstrated a unified, independent standards approach.[27] This line of argument showed how far the AESO/college group had distanced itself from traditional acupuncture rivals.

AESO and the colleges started to widen the campaign against the NH&MRC. They obtained a meeting with the chairperson of the NH&MRC's health care committee, which had commissioned the working party review. The La Trobe Health Sciences dean and the deputy vice chancellor of the University of Technology, Sydney (which was showing some interest in the Sydney college) were also nominated to attend. In advance of the meeting the Melbourne principal wrote to the chairperson: 'Our goal is, we believe, no different to yours, namely to arrive at an outcome which guarantees safe standards of practice of acupuncture in the interests of public health'.[28] The goal was, of course, registration and higher education which, the acupuncturists believed, *were* in the public interest.

A little before the endgame, I obtained approval to have a second look at the health department's working party papers. Amongst them were the minutes of the reconvened working party meeting to consider objections to the first published report.[29] All the pertinent sections had been quoted verbatim, though unattributed, in the minister's letter to the government senator — the one that led acupuncturists to think the next report would remedy the deficiencies of the previous version.

I gave the Melbourne college principal a copy of these minutes in advance of the meeting with the health care committee chairperson. The acupuncturists made much of them: they were used to demonstrate that the working party had agreed the public would be protected from danger by the announcement of safe traditional practitioners but had failed to exercise proper accountability for public safety by not carrying its resolutions into the second published report. Writing to the new federal health minister, the evaluation committee drew attention to the former minister's letter to the senator and to the minutes of the working party meeting and went on to say:

> *In the Working Party's subsequent report (November 1989), this information, crucial to the safety of the Australian public, has been withheld* (emphasis in the original).

> We believe that the Australian public both deserve and have the right to be fully informed about all matters pertaining to their health and that the withholding of such information, especially by a working party of a body constituted to inform the Government and safeguard the public in the area of health, is to be deplored.[30]

The acupuncturists asked the health care committee chairperson to establish another group. It was to identify the role and place of acupuncture in the health care system; identify the educational needs of traditional practitioners to fulfill that role; and to consider support for the establishment of pilot programmes of acupuncture education in New South Wales and Victorian universities.[31] The proposal was that AESO and higher education representatives, the Sydney and Melbourne college principals, and the government senator, be included as members.

They now got their way, though without the senator as a member: the NH&MRC established a further 'Working Party on the Role and Requirements for Acupuncture Education'. It had but one meeting, chaired by the NH&MRC's secretary and attended by two members of the old working party, a senior AMAS practitioner, higher education representatives, the Sydney and Melbourne college principals, the chairman of the Melbourne college board of management (representing the evaluation committee) and an AESO nominee. At last traditional acupuncturists — albeit from only one part of the occupation — had places at the table, and that made all the difference.

With diplomatic nods to the former group, the new working party accepted that acupuncture was currently practised as a primary care modality (that is, a 'technical' way of confining the activity to a limited sphere) and emphasised the need 'to ensure a high standard of safe practice in its continuation' (Loy, 1990). According to the report, desirable relationships between acupuncture practitioners and other health professionals could not be provided by legislation and regulation but the expectation was that 'such relationships would occur as a result of appropriate mutually respectful training programs'. To ensure a high standard of safe acupuncture practice, the 'provision of Acupuncture education in suitably staffed and equipped universities in the tertiary education sector at the undergraduate level' was recommended, along with postgraduate education for other professionals 'interested in providing this modality as part of a range of treatment options'. Reverting to the serious harm argument, and drawing attention to the creation of ACATME, it seemed to the working party that acupuncture had met the West Australian criteria for registration. The three-and-a-quarter-page report concluded with this recommendation: 'In view of the potential dangers inherent in the practice of Acupuncture this Working Party recommends, in the interests of optimal public safety, that the registration of acupuncture practitioners be expedited'.

Further dickering preceded the report going to the NH&MRC (and the registration recommendation was held over to a later meeting).[32] But the course proposals were accepted. The federal department issued a NH&MRC news release which began:

In the interests of providing a high standard of safe acupuncture practice, the National Health and Medical Research Council has recommended the provision of undergraduate acupuncture education in suitably staffed and equipped universities in the tertiary sector.[33]

Against all the odds, this uninfluential but determined coterie of traditional acupuncturists had obtained a measure of official support for their occupation. The NH&MRC was no longer the worst of enemies, whose reports were flawed. A spring to reputability would be made on the authority of its recommendations. The Melbourne college proceeded to announce the fact in seeking the enrollments it desperately needed to survive until La Trobe accepted the course:

Figure 6   College advertisement

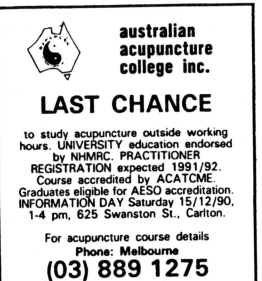

(*The Age, Extra,* p.3. 24 November 1990).

Between the first and second reports of the original working party, its chairman told me:

[Acupuncture] really is a continuing way of treating the psyche with placebos. We do it in another way with drugs. But we do have the probability that our general practitioners have sufficient experience and training to detect any organic diseases. I don't intend to be derogatory but Australian fringe practitioners do not have the anatomical background and medical sciences training to pick up the evolution of organic diseases . . . All these people are seizing on a funny little World Health Organisation report that puts together what a number of people had observed and are turning it into a scientific evidence for acupuncture. That pisses me off no end. And going through the whole business again pisses me off no end . . . I'm not going to advocate registering them — that does not make them more or less lethal . . . Governments tend to do what is quick, expedient and acceptable.

Nevertheless, as a member of the new working party, the chairman of the old one participated in the decision to recommend higher education and registration.

Why did the turnabout occur? Governments were unwilling to proscribe traditional acupuncture — so much was clear — but to recommend government support for it was quite another matter, especially when the body making the recommendation was considered by its opponents to represent the quintessence of reactionary medicine. The traditional acupuncturists reckoned the NH&MRC had been obliged to change tack. 'Obviously they had the riot act read to them', the Melbourne principal commented after the new working party had met. The federal health minister was believed to be supportive and he would have done the reading. There appears to have been some pressure from him, and his predecessor, to resolve a prolonged dispute but no direction to alter the stance taken to that point.

Willis (1989) suggests an altered basis for statutory recognition in what he calls clinical legitimation, meaning recognition that follows on the success of a therapy as demonstrated by its repeated use. But patient acceptance of traditional acupuncture only indirectly bore on the outcome in that the public now had to be protected. Rather than patients being central to legitimation, the widespread adoption of selected alternative therapies by established medical practitioners and their affiliates, like physiotherapists, has been the condition for recognising the groups originally associated with them. Therapies gain reputability by incorporation, which flows back to the promulgating medicines. That is what happened with spinal manipulative therapy and now it had occurred with acupuncture. At no stage did established medical practitioners and physiotherapists say they obtained better results with these therapies than chiropractors, osteopaths and traditional acupuncturists. Instead, the *people* were condemned.

The new working party report did not mention the science of acupuncture (or the lack of it) at all. Danger won the day for traditional acupuncturists. Once there was common ground about the danger of the activity, it followed that all practitioners of it should be made safe. This danger went hand in hand with a recognition of therapeutic potency. The claimed responsibility for patient welfare, on which the established medical repudiation of the alternatives was based, had been turned into support for obligatory higher education and statutory regulation.

ALIGNING WITH SCIENCE

When the fight against the second published working party report was a few months old, the former principal of the Melbourne college published a paper in the acupuncture journal affiliated with AESO and the colleges (Fraser, 1990). It was called 'Two Scientific Frameworks in Acupuncture Research' and sub-titled 'A Review for the Benefit of the Academic Board, La Trobe University, Melbourne'.

Fraser outlined a usual interpretation of the difficulty scientists had in coming to terms with what he called the inexact and poetic language of ancient texts. He expounded a version of the old European doctrine of signatures (see Foucault, 1973, 17-77, for a remarkable account of the seventeenth century transition in thought from resemblances as the categories of knowledge to the analytic representations of identity and difference). Fraser surmised that breaking cell walls with an acupuncture needle might well set off a bioelectric pulse with cells along the acupuncture meridian responding to it. These stable and measurable bioelectric fields could be measured by the use of a machine called the Vega which could be used to test the electromagnetic resonances of homeopathic substances and of points on an acupuncture meridian. Thus, acupuncture could be confirmed and become scientifically acceptable by instrumental verifications of the existence of meridians and points.

The Melbourne principal took exception to the article almost six months after its issue. He wrote to all La Trobe University academic board members to advise them that the college 'in no way endorses either the reference to La Trobe University in the title, nor the views expressed nor the unsubstanciated [sic] claims in the text'.[34] On behalf of the recently formed college board of studies (of which

more in the following chapter), the principal then wrote to Fraser
about his mentioning La Trobe:

> The Board feels that such a reference in the title of an article is
> most unauthodox [sic] and is depremental [sic] to this Colleges'
> efforts to have acupuncture education in Victoria transferred into
> La Trobe University. It is also felt that although you may feel that
> there is some validity to the claims you make in your article, the
> Board feels that such claims are unlikely to have a positive effect on
> the scientific community either inside or outside La Trobe
> University, as these claims are not substanciated [sic] according to
> accepted canons of scientific enquiry.[35]

The college governing body (the committee of management)
followed up with another letter to Fraser. It had considered his
position as patron of the college and his

> use of 'The founder and patron of the Australian Acupuncture
> College in Melbourne, Australia' particularly in relation to your
> above article . . . The Committee of Management unanimously
> supports the view taken by the Board of Studies and the Committee
> unanimously objects to the use of the reference to the A.A.C. and
> your position as a patron when the A.A.C. Inc. is unaware of the
> contents of the article.[36]

The committee went on to say that some uninformed people,
unaware that Fraser had not been involved with the college since he
sold it in 1985 and moved interstate, might mistakenly believe that his
views represented or had the approval of the college. The letter
concluded:

> In future, unless the normal courtesy is extended to the Committee
> of Management of the A.A.C. Inc. to peruse your article and ask the
> present Committee of Management to use your position with the
> present college, the Committee of Management will regretfully
> review your position as patron.

Here was another case of hard-won gains being threatened by
disreputable connections (the new working party had been
established and was about to meet; the college was preparing to re-
submit its course proposal to the La Trobe academic board in the
following year). The college leaders judged the deleterious effects of
Fraser's article by affirming the canons of scientific inquiry, as if
traditional acupuncture itself had already come in from the cold and
had science radiating behind it. However distant he might already be,

Fraser had to submit to control. Those who made difficulties for the cause risked excommunication.

The Melbourne principal spoke of traditional Chinese medicine having an integrated ecological view that was inherent in Chinese culture, not the nineteenth century scientific view that still was common in western medicine. Therefore, he said, it was more likely that western medical science would be incorporated in a traditional Chinese medical view, rather than the reverse. Yet the inclusion of western medical science programmes taught by higher education institutions became a condition for AESO acceptance of other traditional acupuncture courses and the accreditation of their students. Western science, not traditional acupuncture, had come to be the patent for respectability.

Notes

(Unless otherwise noted, documents are from Australian Acupuncture College files).

1. The reports were drafted by a working party which produced three versions, each being final at the time of its presentation: (i) the first, unpublished, was dated 29 March 1988 and circulated with the NH&MRC's health care committee (HCC) agenda for its meeting on 20-21 April 1988 (DCSH files); (ii) after having been sent back for revision, the next version was endorsed by the HCC on 13-14 September 1988, dated 28 September, approved by the full NH&MRC in November and then published (shown in the bibliography as Westerman, 1988); (iii) following further amendment, the third version (n.d.) was endorsed by the HCC on 13-14 September 1989, approved by the full NH&MRC in November and also published (Westerman, 1989).

2. *Acupuncture – Report of the NHMRC Working Party on Acupuncture*, 29 March 1988, p. 59, DCSH files.

3. Recommendations to restrict acupuncture to medical practitioners had been made by earlier NH&MRC reviews (McLeod et al., 1974; Munro-Ashman and Quail, 1979); and by a Victorian Health Advisory Council inquiry (Townsend, 1982) which allowed that other registered practitioners, such as chiropractors and physiotherapists, might also be permitted to use it (Townsend, 1982). Following this last, the state health commission conducted a one year survey of major hospitals and other institutions to discover whether there were cases where acupuncture had caused significant harm. After it, the health minister advised the Melbourne college that there was no reason to hinder the work of acupuncturists in any way because no problems had been reported. Roper, T. (Minister for health) to Fraser, P. (then the college principal), 26 July 1984. In the following year, a federal committee (considering whether national health insurance should be altered to cover services offered by non-medical practitioners) was told by the AMAS that 'the lack of extensive and proper training of non-medical acupuncturists increases considerably the possibility of the spread of serum hepatitis, hepatitis B and more recently AIDS'. Tan, K. (AMAS president) to secretary, Medical Benefits Review Committee, 16 September 1985, AESO files. Having reported this and other criticisms of non-medical acupuncturists in the AMAS submission, and rebuttals of them by AESO, the committee said: 'No evidence was provided to us to support the

AMAS' assertion' (Layton, 1986, 110).

4. McMeekin, J. (acting chairperson, department of physiotherapy) to Scott, J. (La Trobe vice-chancellor), 9 May 1989, Lincoln files.
5. *A Response to the Report of November 1988*, September 1989, p. 2. Zindler, R., for and on behalf of the National Council of the Australian Natural Therapists Association, DCSH files.
6. ANTA's original submission to the working party referred to an 'inexplicable' N.S.W. government decision to accredit the Sydney course and was disparaging about proprietorial control of AESO, which, it said, apparently functioned as a 'rubber stamp to "accredit" students who have undertaken the course conducted by the Acupuncture College (Australia)'. *Submission to Working Party on Acupuncture of N.H. and M.R.C.*, December 1987, pp.33, 43, Australian Natural Therapists Association, DCSH files.
7. ANTA's submission to the working party referred to the natural therapies as having been defined 'as consisting of the four major disciplines of osteopathy, chiropractic, naturopathy and traditional Chinese medicine (TCM) of which acupuncture is an important component'.
8. The reference is to the Australian Acupuncture Association (AAcA), a national traditional acupuncture association but with a large Queensland membership. There had been an attempt to merge AESO with it, which failed (according to AESO leaders) because AAcA was unprepared to submit local colleges to AESO accreditation requirements.
9. AESO was established as part of a proprietary company with unit trust holders (each of whom subscribed $1 000). This had been set up by Jewell, the chiropractor who founded and owned AC(A). The company ran various businesses, including the Sydney college and AESO. Later (1987), AESO obtained statutory appointment as an incorporated association. Its committee comprised the whole: thus the accredited 'members' were not partners in the association and only the subscribers had a say in its management.
10. The Hospitals Contributions Fund, a private insurer, had decided to rebate fees for acupuncture services if guidelines for practitioner recognition could be established. It approached the Sydney college which set up AESO for the purpose in 1977. 'The A.E.S.O. Story – Pioneering Acupuncture in Australia', in *Acupuncture Ethics and Standards Organisation – A Practitioner's Guide*, (1987). At first, the idea was that rebates would be paid for acupuncture services referred by registered medical practitioners. According to a Sydney college student essay (Vollmer, A. 'The History of the Acupuncture Ethics and Standards Organization', 19 October 1988), an account which staff present at the time endorsed, the N.S.W. branch of the AMA opposed medical referrals to unlicensed traditional acupuncturists and the insurance fund then allowed reimbursement for direct services.
11. Berle, C. (for AESO board of governors) to Zindler, R., 16 August 1983. All AESO practitioners were later told they would have to formally sign an undertaking to abide by the new provision when renewing their accreditation for 1984. Jewell, H. (for AESO) in a circular letter, 6 September 1983, AESO files.
12. 'Addition to the A.E.S.O. Code of Ethics Article VI. Section 6', (1983). Subsequently incorporated as section 1.12 in the 1989 version of the code. AESO files.
13. Circular letter to other colleges by Berle, C. (secretary to AESO board of governors), 2 September 1986; and AESO's *Accreditation Guidelines – Current as of 1st January 1989*, n.d. (1989). AESO files.
14. Zindler, R. (ANTA executive director and vice president) to Berle, C., 13 September 1989, AESO files.

15. Spicer, M. (executive officer, Sydney College of Natural Therapies and Traditional Chinese Medicine) to Rogers, C., (the AC(A) principal), 10 July 1989.
16. Rogers to Spicer, 28 July 1989.
17. Taylor, I. (Minister for Health) to Berle, C. (AESO Secretary), 17 June 1987, AESO files.
18. 'Review of the Status of Unregistered Health Occupation Groups — The Committee Report to the Minister of Health for Western Australia', September 1989, pp. 9-10, Legislation Review and Development Branch, Health Department of Western Australia.
19. 'Response of the A.E.S.O. Federal Executive to the Review of the Status of Unregistered Health Occupation Groups Prepared for the Minister for Health for Western Australia in September 1989', November 1989, p. 4.
20. 'Discussion Paper on the Statutory Regulation of Health Practitioner Groups', January 1990. Circulated by the N.S.W. minister for health.
21. The evaluation committee's report of the meeting was published in the journal associated with AESO and the colleges: 'Report on the Meeting between Dr. Neal Blewett and Representatives of the Traditional Acupuncture Profession to Discuss Major Flaws in the Current National Health and Medical Research Council's Report on Acupuncture', *Australian Journal of Traditional Chinese Medicine 4*, 4 (May 1989), pp. 5-8
22. The minister's private secretary told me later that the working party had not been outside the minister's office. Three of the four working party members lived in Melbourne, and one of them had used acupuncture in his general practice, but none of the traditional acupuncturists had ever met members.
23. Blewett, N. (Minister for community services and health) to Zakharov, O., 28 June 1989.
24. Watson, K. (as Victorian co-ordinator of the evaluation committee) to Blewett, N., 17 February 1990.
25. Blewett, N. to Watson, K., 8 March 1990.
26. Blewett, N. to Batten, H., 3 April 1990. Lincoln files.
27. In the compendious response to the second working party report: 'Critique of the Revised (November 1989) National Health and Medical Research Council's Working Party Report on Acupuncture — Prepared by the Committee for the Evaluation of the NH&MRC Working Party's Report on Acupuncture', 1990, pp. 54-63. Lincoln files.
28. Watson, K. (as Victorian co-ordinator of the evaluation committee) to Horvath, D. (chairperson of the HCC), 24 April 1990.
29. 'Report of Meeting, Working Party on Acupuncture', 26 May 1989, DCSH files.
30. Watson, K. (as Victorian co-ordinator) to Howe, B. (Minister for Community Services and Health), 16 May 1990.
31. As confirmed in a letter after the meeting: Watson, K. (as Victorian co-ordinator) to Horvath, D., 16 May 1990.
32. This recommendation, which the NH&MRC's health care committee did not endorse but did not reject, has been in hot dispute.
33. News Release: 'Acupuncture: Role and Requirements for Education', National Health and Medical Research Council, 9 November 1990.
34. Watson, K. to La Trobe academic board members, 13 August 1990. Lincoln files.
35. Watson, K. (for the board of studies) to Fraser, P., 14 August 1990.
36. Hobbs, G. (for the committee of management) to Fraser, P., 19 September 1990.

VI

THE PURGE

We used to be a very close group who got on well together and shared a lot.

(Principal of the Melbourne acupuncture college.)

CHANGING THE COLLEGE STRUCTURE

The acupuncturists had been battling for over a year to counter the NH&MRC. New staff and students were ready supporters but the old guard carried the fight. As mentioned earlier, at the start of 1989, six of the thirty students who had just completed the course were picked out to join the staff. Some were about to go to Beijing for a three-month hospital internship and would teach on their return. Others were to begin lecturing and tutoring right away. Transferring the course to La Trobe University was of paramount importance at a staff 'retreat' held shortly after the graduation. Teaching and assessment procedures were to be reformulated on the university model.

In a conversation over lunch, there was general agreement that moving to La Trobe University would bring on many alterations to the course. One teacher noted that change had happened already, as instanced by the introduction of western medical subjects taught by the Lincoln Institute of Health Sciences. Another remarked that he did not teach acupuncture as he had done. The students would not let him — their expectations had altered. What next? There was a difference in emphasis rather than a division. On one side, the conviction was that as part of a university the task was to systematically investigate acupuncture and to report on it in the literature. One of the new staff countered by saying that Chinese medicine was an empirical science: look at the Shanghai techniques, they were entirely about results! The clinical application of acupuncture should not be sacrificed to theorising and academic publishing. Other new staff shared that view.

Twelve months later, three of the new staff, along with an old-stager, faced proceedings to remove them from teaching in the programme. Immediately before these events, one of the senior teachers told me there were divisions within the college:

> There is some dispute now, people getting together in corners, wanting to bring on the revolution, the young ones . . . It's *so* like the situation I've seen in [secondary] schools. The trouble with leadership is that you are so alone: you need to have five or six heads about you and a board for support.

The board he was talking about was the group that managed the college. There were thirteen members, or subscribers, to an incorporated association and they elected seven of their number to a committee of directors. In a sense, the members *were* the college. From time to time there would be references to 'our' college, distinguishing those who were members from those teachers who were not. They were all joined in the cause represented by the college but the separation of owners from employees (though many of the owners were also employees) was there and could be raised in the course of disputes.

The principal had had his difficulties with three of the seven directors. Since they were not directly associated with teaching the course they were called outside members. Two were graduates of the college and the third, married to one of them, was a lawyer. The principal resented the outside members not accepting his recommendations and the tight control of finances exercised by the one who acted as treasurer. He believed an erosion of confidence in him had been promoted by the former college administrator (a salaried employee) and by a former teacher who had been upset when her teaching engagement was reduced following student complaints. The principal maintained the two had 'got at' several of the outside directors who subsequently questioned his recommendations.

The principal had sought earlier to introduce an intermediate steering group (following the example set by his Sydney equivalent) but the outside directors had rejected it. This time matters came to a head over pay scales. Teachers received hourly rates which were significantly below those for casual university staff and an attempt was made to adjust them by more than the usual annual inflationary variation. The change had been opposed by the treasurer who, so the principal said, had maintained that the teachers 'would not be able to get academic appointments any rate'. Resentment over the payment issue provoked support for management changes. The principal and the unit co-ordinators — staff designated to manage sections of the course — held meetings where anger about the rejection of salary increases (inflamed by the treasurer's reported comment) was mixed with the principal's annoyance about being impeded by the outside directors. As a co-ordinator said to the principal at the first of these meetings:

> You were talking about your frustrations. I thought it was unreasonable the situation you were in. The way it came across to me, you were dealing with issues then you had to go to the board and it was decided over again. To me, it seemed wrong. The board appoints a principal then he goes about his job. The individual issues should be decided by the principal. Otherwise it is undermining his job. The only way I could see out of that is perhaps bringing in another level of people fully involved with the college instead of taking things to the board.

The outside directors were considered to be 'out of touch' with the college. This co-ordinator (who was also a member of the college association) saw it as a structural rather than a personal problem: the board had been part and parcel of the college in the early days but now the outside directors had become distant from the college as it had grown and the role of the board had become inappropriate. Nonetheless, the dispute kept getting back to the miserly attitude that the outside directors had taken over pay. The co-ordinators spoke at length about their commitment of time and energy to the college. The cause was still the cause, they did not complain about the effort, but employment should be adequately remunerated. If there was no money then there was no answer, one said. But the money was there — the college had reserves which the treasurer had invested — and that, as another said, was 'salt in the wound'.

At their second meeting, the principal explained:

> The cynical reason they [the outside directors] refused to put up the fees was that they thought we wouldn't get jobs in the tertiary sector any rate. A person who can think like that about the college and the staff has a very dim view about the college and its future.

The co-ordinator who had suggested the need for a structural alteration took that up: 'Anyone who knew where we were going *never* would make a statement belittling our staff!'. The principal followed on: the college was approaching the critical stage in its struggle to get into La Trobe; the staff had to be helped to prepare for the transfer; the battle against the NH&MRC was reaching its peak:

> It's our last bloody chance! The last thing I need is an obstructive board, a board I have to fight and battle. They should not have a say. If it means getting rid of people so the next few months run like clockwork then I don't care if they go.

The principal and the three other directors who were staff members formulated a proposal which gave authority for college management to a new body, an executive committee with the principal in the chair and unit co-ordinators as members.[1] It was a classic division. While the directors retained overall responsibility for the college (which was their statutory obligation), the executive obtained control of 'day-to-day' activities and would act as the principal's advisory committee. He was 'charged with the ultimate authority over day-to-day matters of both an academic and an administrative nature', and was 'responsible for the appointment of academic staff in consultation with the Executive Committee'. A financial management procedure gave the new college administrator greater control over money. A concurrent proposal, signed by the same four inside members, recommended immediate pay increases to levels which approximated university rates.[2] These recommendations might well have resulted in a split between the four signatories and the three outside directors but the principal was past bothering. The other teachers were more concerned that they stay and, after some discomfort, the proposals were accepted and the outside directors remained.

In the eventual structure, the directors became a committee of management and the six unit co-ordinators (including the principal) became a board of studies with the additional power to decide on academic direction and curriculum matters.[3] This result consolidated the influence of the principal.

DEALING WITH DISLOYALTY

The principal soon used the new board of studies. There had been a number of difficulties over the second half of 1989, which centred on the teaching of point location (the places for needle insertion). A letter from the principal to all teachers, signed on his behalf by one of the senior staff who was dean of students, drew attention to reports of first-year student concern about alleged staff disagreements over the correct location of specific points.[4] The students were said to be further distressed by one or more teachers telling the class that the location of points in the prescribed text, written by the principal of the Sydney college, were incorrect. The letter went on to note that the text was stipulated by the college for the purposes of teaching, learning and assessment. While the possibility of more than one opinion was allowed:

> it is not appropriate for staff members to have disagreements about these matters in front of students. Furthermore, to be so presumptuous as to claim that the locations given in Dr. Rogers' book are incorrect, with the inference that you know better, is both arrogant and totally unacceptable. To experienced practitioners, T.C.M. is an art as well as a science and, as an art, leaves room for differences of approach and opinion.
>
> I can only presume that the person, or persons, concerned regard their beginner's knowledge of T.C.M. as superior to Dr. Rogers' experience and knowledge gained through 15 years of teaching and practice.
>
> The staff responsible have caused confusion and a degree of distress to the first year students. Unless they learn to exercise professional behaviour, humility and respect for their fellow staff members and colleagues they will not be welcome to continue working at the college.

This warning was directed at some of the new staff, two of whom had returned from Beijing and were involved in point location teaching. The difference seemed to turn on a technical matter and on the need for teaching conformity but the heaviness of the letter, and the formality, suggested larger issues were at stake.

The teachers were appointed from year to year. At the end of 1989, the principal summoned four of them before the board of studies 'to discuss some serious allegations that have been brought to our attention'.[5] The provoking incident was an evening discussion arranged by some of the staff. One who attended had told the principal that others at the meeting 'want to take the college over; they want to take over the barracks and burn the flag'. The principal explained his position to me:

> First and foremost, it's the loyalty of staff to each other that counts. After that, the quality of teaching and their interaction with the

students. It's impossible if you can't have loyalty: how can you have a college where people are saying libellous things, outrageous things about other staff and about graduates? They think because they went to China they know *everything*.

The principal had a range of complaints about the four (only two of whom had been to China for their internship). He was convinced all his evidence demonstrated the undesirability of keeping them on. Immediately before the new board of studies met to interview the first two, the principal laid out the case he intended to present to four of the five board members over lunch. Supposedly, each of the staff was attending a job interview: the committee of management had given the board the right to determine employment and that was what had to be decided. The charges amounted to active conspiracy to overthrow college structures and processes, 'badmouthing' the college by questioning its standards, criticising its administration, being absolutist and dictatorial in class, disputing in front of students. The combination was different from one to the next but the common element was their meeting together to take over the barracks and burn the flag. The two who thought 'that because they have been to China know everything' came in for some attention. As one of the board of studies members said in the course of this discussion 'You'd think they'd have learnt their lesson in China. They were right near the square [i.e. Tien An Minh Square]. You have a perfect right to demonstrate – until the leadership decides that you shouldn't'. He went on to speak of 'the lesson of Tien An Minh Square', referring to the military suppression of student demonstrators there in June of the previous year, when the party of acupuncture college graduates had been in Beijing on their hospital internship.

The principal said to his colleagues 'They have a right to complain but we have the right to decide who is employed and the question is whether we want them teaching when we know what they have been actively seeking to do'. He had a number of reports about meetings to overturn the college organisation; he felt the evidence was overwhelming that there had been 'active attempts to plan the overthrow of the college structure'.

One of the board of studies members said: 'It's not really a job interview is it?' So far as he knew, one of the four had a good teaching reputation with the students. The principal had heard otherwise but, he said,

That's not the point; we are not really considering their *teaching* ability; it's their badmouthing of college people, standards of the course, the theses especially, *and* their seeking to overthrow the structures. The point is, do we want to continue to employ people when we know that what they do is use paid time to criticise the college to students and undermine staff relationships? . . . We have to be clear that this is not a court of law. Their contracts have expired and we have to decide who we hire to teach in 1990.

However, the principal did agree to take out the reference to job interviews in his script. The board members proceeded to talk about changing the locks. All the student addresses were in the office and it had to be faced that one of the things the four could do was write to all the students. They would have to ask for their keys back but that was not possible because they still had to make a decision. They would ask for them later that evening. The board returned from lunch and trooped into the back room to begin the interviews.

After the interviews, members said they were sure about the first of the accused to appear. He had denied everything, including a meeting. But the second had showed that up by agreeing there had been a meeting and by saying that two of the others (including the first person interviewed) had organised it. The charge against the first was immediately diverted to one of deception. As the principal said later 'When [the second person interviewed] came in and agreed that there had been a meeting, that was it, people were saying "I can't work with [the first] after that. He told us an untruth"'.

The charge against the second underwent a similar translation. Amongst other things, he was said to have intended needling one inch deep on a point to the side of the eye socket but had been physically stopped by another staff member. The principal commented that the teacher had actually boasted to him about this; what he had wanted to do was 'incredibly dangerous'. The teacher was later cleared on this charge: the person who was supposed to have stopped him reported that he had not tried to needle but had only said that this was the way they did it in China in order to get the Qi and that if one didn't go so deep then one needn't bother using the point at all. The principal said that indicated the charged teacher had not told him the truth. At a second meeting with the board, this teacher said he had been misinterpreted, misunderstood and taken out of context, which meant, as the principal said afterwards, he had a communication problem and *that* was not good for his teaching.

The denials only confirmed the reality of the problem and the wisdom of removing the cause. In rejecting the charge that there had been a plot, one of the people interviewed said that she had never heard of any such thing until a fourth-year college student had asked at a party: 'When is the coup?'. While this was intended to demonstrate to the board that the meeting had not been concerned to formulate such a plan, the mention of a coup had the opposite effect. The principal told me: 'I didn't pursue it but I said, "All you've done is give us another source that confirms there was an aim"'. Later, he returned to the topic:

> We were quite shocked that the fourth year student should have been asking 'When is the coup?' That party was several months ago — it means that the attitudes must have been there then, the issues must have been discussed. It's difficult. Six years ago there were only two teachers, me and [the then principal]. 1989 was the year when we had the biggest number of staff aboard. And a lot of them are junior staff. I don't mean *they* are junior, they might have done a lot of [school] teaching but they have not had a lot of experience with traditional Chinese medicine. Their heads are too big. Well, they made their ploy, their grab at power. Sometimes they succeed, but this time they got the chop. I feel comfortable with the result.

Two of the staff were not renewed. The two who had been to China were put on a form of probation. One of them, who had written before being interviewed to ask for a detailing of the allegations and their source and had not received a reply, was allowed a small number of classes but had reasons for not teaching in the first semester. The board felt that this teacher might not have been so directly engaged in plotting. The other, who was not given any teaching, was expected to undergo a rehabilitation process by attending staff in-service events. His failure to do so was said to indicate that he had not given leaders 'any opportunity to show us his engagement'. But as one of the students put it: 'He is not going to "suck bums", to quote him!'. These two had been effectively shut out. The principal did not want them back.

Different complaints had been raised against each of the four. For example, some months earlier one was said to have presumptuously thrust himself forward by 'demanding' the right to review the curriculum (he was said to have been told by the principal, 'It's none of your business, it's not *your* college'). Another (formerly a senior teacher and unit co-ordinator) had withdrawn the level of visible commitment and presence demanded of him. The two who had been to China had been disruptive to staff and students. These people were, as the principal repeatedly maintained, rabid, fanatical, overbearing, big-headed and disruptive. After a board interview with one of them, the principal said:

> He didn't see that he was any of these things but people felt intimidated when working with him. What he doesn't see is that they would feel just as intimidated when asked [by him] if they *were* intimidated.

The removal of teachers who were thought to stand against college purposes had its effect on those who remained. As a staff member commented to me:

> Let's face it, [the principal] has got his way with [the creation of] the board of studies and had put his own people on it. Now he is the moving force over the removal of these lecturers. It's a message to me to be cautious.

Others also demonstrated that they had learned the lesson. The marking of fourth-year student research projects was a sensitive topic because a charge against one of the sacked teachers was that he had told the college administrator that many of the theses had been poor and had not deserved to pass (he was accused of denigrating his colleagues and college standards). During a later staff discussion about thesis assessment, one teacher disagreed with the suggested marking distribution: he said that at least 50% should be allocated for thesis content. The principal flared up. It was not only a matter of doing research well but of structuring and presenting it well. The teacher backed away saying, 'The job of the college is to pass on content. I believe in cabinet solidarity but I believe views ought to be put! I've raised it, but if all are happy with it as it is . . .'

There was a silence. '*Some* of us aren't happy', one of the senior figures interposed, referring to the argument this teacher had been putting. 'That's O. K.', he replied, 'I believe in cabinet solidarity'.

THE MESSAGE FROM CHINA

Despite the principal's unquenchable optimism, the future looked bleak at the time staff were being charged. The college had failed to gain admission to La Trobe University and no progress had been made in the dispute with the NH&MRC. Enrollments for first year were down by half to fifteen, which led to difficulties in financing the operation. The principal was embattled. He believed he had evidence of an internal plan to drag the college down, to confound all it stood for.

What really condemned the four, one of the principal's informants told me, was that they were expressing their disagreement to students — 'sowing dissension amongst students'. Students had to be protected. Their 'distress' had been mentioned earlier in relation to the point location classes and similar comments were made during the proceedings.

When teaching recommenced the following year, many of those in the second-year class talked a great deal about the departure of the two who had been to China, which they believed was a great loss. One explained:

> What they brought back from China was something very different. They brought a precision to it, an accuracy. They replaced art with science. I had no particular reason to like them. Before they came back I'd been getting nine out of ten [in tests], then I got six out of ten! I thought: hey, what's this? Then I realised they were far more precise, rigorous. A lot of the students go to them [for treatment]. The old guard in the college doesn't appreciate the need for accuracy. It's entirely a political matter. They are being pushed out.

The students present agreed with this. Another said:

> These people were an inspiration to me! I mean, they [the college leaders] are into stagnation — that's not what acupuncture is all about! It's an autocracy that's frightened of change. I mean, it's not as if they were going to overturn the college or anything — they just wanted to make things different and the autocracy was resisting any change.

There was a shared fear that if they raised the sackings as an issue then they would be singled out for retribution. They had heard about students complaining some years earlier and many being failed. One student was said to have been disciplined for standing up to the college. These stories were believed: if you got out of line the college was likely to punish you. That led to a catalogue of resentments about the college. They wondered where the college money, their money, went. They thought the principal had become too detached from the college by his campaign against the government. He was a good teacher but he was out of touch with the *clinical* situation, with practice. They picked up on NH&MRC criticisms about the qualifications of acupuncture teachers.

Disaffection had set in amongst this group of students. Even the cause of university admission was viewed sceptically. One second-year student said to another:

> The college is always talking about when acupuncture is at La Trobe and the course is registered. But what happens when something goes that way? It cuts off some of the knowledge, leads to it being regular knowledge and some of the rest which is experimental but important is cut off. It authorises the old men in power.

A few teachers also had their reservations. One said that while the principal was an excellent man for the times, politically, he was not the fount of all wisdom about acupuncture:

> As to the sacked staff, we can ill afford to do without them, we need a resource of good people. People may not realise the enormous competence they gained in China. They might have come back a bit full of themselves but they carried a great deal of value. They might have gone about it the wrong way but they needed to be kept.

Right from this teacher's own first year in the college, there had been 'an underlying ferment' about the quality of teaching and about professional competency. What the people who had been to China brought back was considerable competency.

What, on the one side, was seen as disruption and an insufferable conceit, was, on the other, an affirmation of the pre-eminence of clinical knowledge and performance. The four wanted to improve the course. They all denied any plan to stage a coup. One told me that the letter they had received (about not disputing college texts) had been the start of it: 'That was what the meeting was all about, that a letter like that could be sent out to all staff.' The teacher who attended the meeting and spoke to the principal about taking over the barracks and burning the flag had the same interpretation. He told me:

> It was an intemperate letter . . . The long and short of it was that everyone was peeved when they got this letter. That was the sort of thing that got things going . . . It was a crucial letter. It was an insult to the people who had been to China. They probably thought in their naivety that they were going to smarten the college up. It was

just a communication problem, that's all. It could have been solved at a staff meeting.

Another of those sacked said to me that it was ridiculous to suggest they were plotting: 'We were talking together as friends. We didn't have any other intention than to seek changes'. About the two who had been to China, this teacher said:

> That had a great effect on them. They'd been in the presence of God and they'd come back with the Gospel. Of course, they are accused of being zealots — I agree with that — but they had heard the true gospel and they were enthused. The students were inspired by it.

The way that one who had been to China put it was:

> We saw a lot of things that were incredibly useful. When we went there we were laughed at. It's not that our knowledge was poor — our course was good — but we really knew very little about needle technique and point location, and the turning of information rapidly into diagnosis. Acupuncture becomes a precise science when you see the way the Chinese do it. The truth is that you feel happy about it. We learned to be completely *au fait* with our information, to use it and to know that it works. You realise the importance of precise point location, the finesse of it. Taoism is pretty messy but acupuncture is a precise science.

That led to a criticism of the college leaders:

> They are doing no clinical work. There are no options for clinical work. Until they do, they are turning out inferior practitioners because they don't know how to put a needle in . . . It's a joke, a farce, the students simply aren't getting the quantity or the quality of clinical experience. The four hundred hour bit [i.e. the clinical practicum requirement] is absurd. Any medical committee would see that it's absolutely insufficient, especially when it's mainly observation — the practitioner doesn't want you to stick needles in his patients.

The principal argued that the college was doing the best it could with its limited funds and lack of access to hospitals. Besides, there were only a few AESO accredited practitioners who took students — about fourteen of them. While leaders blamed the profession for its apathy and lack of support for the college, the sacked teacher thought the leaders could do much more. The college premises ought to be used for a student clinic which could 'get in the poor, you know, $2 a treatment if you are a pensioner or $5 if you have a health card. Soon the politicians would be saying, "there they are, treating the poor and the old and getting good results"!' The problem was, he continued, that the college had been concentrating on one thing, the NH&MRC:

You really need two wings that communicate with each other. One is fantastically keen about getting registration and the other is softer and supportive and directed to encouraging the practitioners . . . A lot of people out there who are really good are pissed off [with the college]. The end result is the alienation of the profession from the college. It's as if you are continually backing yourself into a corner, becoming more isolated, while you keep saying, 'We're winning! We're winning!'

The second graduate to have gone to China said: 'Remember, we'd just been students and our priorities came from the way students like to be treated, not power within a structure. We were on about communication'. Like the others, this teacher was deeply upset about the way the board interviews were conducted: 'The whole tone was: "you've done something really evil and we're telling you why we can't employ you"'. The purge in China and that in the college were bitter experiences and they were somehow linked. Both had to do with suppression and the exercise of power, and with more than that: being falsely accused and yet in an inexplicable way being responsible for the outcome.

It was so unfair, it came out as if [one of those dismissed] was responsible for the whole thing which was completely untrue. He drove me up there and actually said on the way: 'Look, I want to be teaching in that college next year and I don't want to get involved in anything that will stop that' . . . China was a shocking experience in the end. When this happened in the college I felt really kicked in the guts, I felt too hurt. The day before [the Tien An Minh Square shootings] the Australians went to the square to express solidarity and the groups parted to let them through. That night the radio blamed foreign devils for provoking one million people to strike. I was in my room when the massacre started and my room-mate was actually in the square being fired at. He came back at 4 a.m. with a graze on his cheek. Then we are told, all the Australians must get out, the army is going to purge the students. They came and fired on the college for six hours. They were single shots, aimed shots. You put all these thoughts together: you're supposed to have incited one million people to strike; they were going to come and get us. You realise that kidneys control the lower Yin – I had diarrhoea. The ironic thing is that [the room-mate in Beijing] was going to be at that meeting to talk about AESO and the NH&MRC Report. Had he made it we would have been less concerned about discussing other things . . . I feel f . . . by what they've done to me.

LOYALTY – AND SURVIVAL

When the college ran its next in-service seminar, a year after the first, a session was devoted to college structures. The principal explained that the new board of studies had come about because people had taken of a lot more responsibility from the days when he and two of the others present were the sole teachers. The staff broke into three groups to discuss the elements of responsibility of teachers. When they came back to a plenary session, loyalty and working together as a team figured in all three reports. The principal commented:

Remember the college is nothing other than us that are here now . . . Our aim is to heal, not only in health but rifts in the college. Bring them to attention before they turn into a chronic disease – that refers to loyalty.

The academic from another institution who was hired to run in-service programmes also conducted a new students orientation weekend that year. In one exercise, staff and students paired off and one with eyes open led the other around with eyes closed. They returned and sat in a circle. The organiser invited them to discuss what it felt like to be led and to lead. After various testimonies, he summarised: 'Obviously this whole thing is about trust and responsibility to each other'. A student agreed: 'If we can emanate a feeling of trust to patients, they will be reliant on you'. The organiser emphasised that students had to trust their lecturers; and that lecturers had to be trustworthy. 'Create an environment that is comfortable and trusting', he concluded. The principal drove the message home:

Because it is easy for people to fragment into clubs or cliques, we have to put that aside in order to learn TCM . . . If people know each other and know they can trust each other – any group of people together, going through a course like this – need to lend advice together.

Those who got into trouble with the college considered that they were punished for becoming *too* loyal — to the cause of Chinese medicine — which led to their being charged with fanaticism. As those who had been to China saw it (and they by no means agreed about technique), their approaches introduced precision. One said: 'It's the immediate recognition of point location and all the other things — depth, angle, needle type — that's what we learned, and it really worked!' And later:

> They call this fanatical and a doctrinal blue but our rigour came from a belief that if a needle is to go into the body with a minimum of trauma then you'll have to put it in with the greatest skill . . . If you are just off, then you have to poke it around before you find the Qi.

The four took a firm stance. One spoke about making sure 'from the beginning that we only learn TCM and so not confuse it with western terms . . . When you are doing TCM you should stick to TCM diagnosis'. They rather shared the opinion of the working party about standards. Another was annoyed about the mystics 'who go on about the ineffability and numinosity of TCM — spare us from them! A lot of it sounds heavy new age, which makes me want to throw up. It's been hi-jacked by hippies!'.

The course was to be renewed and transformed by going back to the high authority of the ancient texts and the practices of contemporary Chinese exponents. But that could be seen by some to be doctrinaire. The coup idea went together with this fanaticism and was taken to be a political expression of it. What was promoted as a revival, a return to the true practice of this medicine, was taken by the principal to be a subversion of the institution that stood for it. Yet only the principal believed a coup was being formulated. Other board members were unconvinced. A key office-holder (the teacher who chaired the committee of directors and was a member of the board of studies) told me afterwards: 'That was not my personal concern at all. There was no clear evidence of a coup being planned'. In fact, it was not possible: none of the four was a member of the college association and all but one of the board of studies members were subscribers. The four had no staff backing, only the enthusiasm of many of their students.

ANOTHER ORGANISATION?

By the cumulation of allegations against them, the four, who did not constitute a group at all, had been made into one by their supposedly joint purpose: the intended subversion of college organisation. The board identified them as a faction by their collective failure to meet loyalty expectations. Beforehand, they were part of a loose circle of friends with some complaints about the leadership being out of touch (just what the leaders thought about the outside directors). After their expulsion, the four did indeed become enemies of the college. They had an abiding sense of resentment and injustice in common.

Along with other college graduates who shared their disaffection, they began to coalesce into an association whose purposes were defined by all the things the college was not. At the end of my stay with the acupuncturists, these outsiders held a meeting which was largely taken up with condemnations of the college leadership. Some wanted to align with another organisation called Access TCM Australia. One of the sacked teachers had told me earlier that this body had itself resulted from practitioner dissatisfactions and was made up of people 'who are genuinely democratic, who are not into that [power] game, who are sharing'. At the meeting he told the others: 'All bullshit has to go! If we got together behind Access TCM, then forget all the bullshit!'. They heard the college was in a deep financial crisis. The treasurer had invested the reserves in a building society that had crashed and a special mid-year intake had failed to attract additional students. The college would fold as it deserved, and a good thing too, because of the things 'they' had done.

One of the college graduates (who emerged as the respected voice of the meeting) suggested another approach:

> You can't take negative actions to any advantage . . . If we set up something totally credible then it will grow . . . It's a lot of work, a lot of energy, it's two years down the road. The last thing we want to see is factionalising.

They needed to set up a constructive alternative to the college, 'not something in opposition to it', she said. Of course, it would be seen by the college management to be just that and others at the meeting wanted it to be so but their aim was diverted. The group hovered on the edge of wanting to work within by attracting a block of AESO practitioner support but the new organisation won out: 'It's great, very Chinese, very communist, I love it!', said another college graduate. They discussed a title and came up eventually with 'TCM Action', then 'Working Group' was added.

Their spokesperson stressed it had to do with broad-based community education. They agreed that they had to get incorporated, though the supporter of communistic enterprise did not like it: 'I'm against all that organisation bullshit!'. The aims were listed: community education; information clearing house; practitioner network; student support; balance of clinical and practical versus theoretical education; to refer, inform, advise. 'And research' someone added. Yes, they agreed, and research. They would meet again in a month. 'We want to finalise some sort of organisation that has this sort of charter', the new leader said. Chinese medicine, the true article, had to be preserved and made known. It was a tentative movement within the movement, an inward reaction to the college and AESO which (like Molloy's Chiropractic Society of Australia) had an outwardly-directed community-education platform.

In its turn, the college board had been defined by the actions of the four. In rejecting them the board confirmed that it was the college organisation. As Erikson has said (1966, 13):

Each time the community moves to censure some act of deviation . . . and convenes a formal ceremony to deal with the responsible offender, it sharpens the authority of the violated norm and restates where the boundaries of the group are located.

Individually, board members were distressed by what had happened. 'The whole thing', one said, 'was intensely discomforting and unpleasant. I mean, they were colleagues'. But the board itself became an effective group as a result of this settlement. When the principal said (on many subsequent occasions) that it was not *his* decision but that of the board he re-affirmed board solidarity around him.

Thereafter, the board was clearly the group that managed the college. Loyalty to the idea of Chinese medicine fused with loyalty to the institution. The cause it represented was also defined by external opposition. As the principal said to the assembled students (who had been called together to hear the bad news about belt-tightening, including a 12.5% cut in staff payment rates, following the building society crash):

The first thing I want to mention [is] Why course accreditation? Why registration? Ever since acupuncture has been practised in Australia there has been a threat hanging over it. That threat is the medical profession. The only way to protect the integrity of traditional acupuncture is to claim it first . . . Unless you fight, you die.

CONSOLIDATING AUTHORITY

To use Weber's distinction between communal and associative orientations to social action (1978, 40-43), the college had shifted away from an affectual relation to one marked by its rationalised mode of social organisation. It was a matter of emphasis: Weber noted that the great majority of social relationships were communal to some degree and at the same time determined by associative factors. Individuals continued to be joined by their faith in traditional acupuncture but the new structure now more closely defined the way in which the cause was to be maintained and prosecuted.

The prospect of transfer to the university had sharpened interest in and competition for academic careers in traditional acupuncture. There had been a good deal of jockeying for position. A segment had consolidated — 'the senior corps', as the chairperson of the committee of management (the directors) called it in identifying them as board of studies members. Thus the board gave expression to a staff partition which combined loyalty, management prerogatives, and access to future rewards. Appeals might still be made to the band of friends of traditional acupuncture — the college that was nothing but its staff — but it had taken on a tighter, more differentiated structure. It was less an organised totality of beliefs and more, in Durkheim's analogy with the living body (1964, 130-131), an organic college solidarity.

According to the usual interpretation of its subjective meaning, the communal type of relationship was, Weber said (1978, 42), the most radical antithesis of conflict. Again, it was a matter of emphasis: there had been many previous conflicts in the college, and fractious students had been disciplined. But the differences over pay and loyalty and the race for university employment both sharpened the membership boundary *and* extended formalisations and distances in the social relations of staff. The college acted against the four staff in a very official way. Their arraignment before the board and the reading out of charges could not have been more unlike an informal settlement. The reaction to it showed just how mistaken these staff were in supposing they belonged to an equal company of like-minded enthusiasts. One said to me about the summons to appear before the board to answer serious allegations: 'This was a letter I had to sign for [i.e., it had been sent by certified mail]. That really got to me'. Another told me:

> When I got in there [to the board meeting] it's absurd, wrong. You've got [the principal] reading from notes — 'you did this, you did that' — an inquisition, a whole lot of allegations collected together from odd bits; and then when they can't prove a damn thing they get onto the personal stuff: 'you've been fanatical, become a zealot since you went to China!'

As Becker and his colleagues found in their study of medical education, the major divisions in the hierarchical organisation of the hospital were legitimated by increasing degrees of clinical experience (H.S. Becker et al., 1961, 234-235). Noting the constant recourse to this authority to settle points during a case conference, one of the observers in this study commented: 'This is a lovely subordinating device in relation to the students and the house staff . . . Logic or reason really don't enter into it; it's just a matter of experience and naturally the older men have had a lot of experience'. In the acupuncture college a different sort of clinical experience, that obtained by the two of the four who had been in China, emerged as a contender. A shadow was cast on the status owing to leaders. The immediate response was a blunt letter to all staff which drew attention to the presumption of beginners.

The legitimacy of the board of studies was held to reside in the superior knowledge and experience of its members as well as in its formal powers. While the college itself might have been thought to be under threat, at least by the principal, the reform purpose of the four staff — their wanting to get back to the true practice of traditional acupuncture — amounted to an explicit criticism. The rightful ascendancy of the leading teachers was being questioned on substantive grounds: the presumption consisted in advocating other ways to teach the course.

The Chinese leadership had found that even when politically significant elements demonstrated the withdrawal of due regard, the control of office remained and could be translated into enforcement of the formal order if used quickly. There, dissidence was characterised as subversion and blamed on the moral failings of the demonstrators in Tien An Minh Square. The principal had emphasised two grounds for dismissing the four: (i) their plot to take over the barracks and burn the flag; (ii) their disloyalty to the college and to colleagues. Each of the four had exhibited deficiencies as members of the social group by making derogatory remarks (and additionally in one case, by withdrawal from normal intercourse with other staff). Such charges might be deflected but out of them arose what was the key shortcoming, so far as the majority of board of studies members were concerned. Their 'letting us down by lying to us' enabled the decision to discard three of them to be made. The moral touchstone for continued assembly was that people who gave each other due honour evidenced it by trustworthiness. They just could not be trusted any more.

As we have seen (in chapter 3) a quadrant typology has been used to chart the movement of a Trotskyist party (Rayner, 1986) and the Salvation Army (Robertson, 1972). Rayner found that the sequence of change was important:

> Only by developing a strong group boundary, and appropriating control over it through witch-hunts and expulsions, and high membership turnover was [the leader] able to consolidate his pre-eminent position, and institute a fully bureaucratic system (1986, 66).

In the acupuncture college, the group boundary was consolidated by the money issue. The principal had been complaining for quite some time that three of the directors regularly checked his proposals. But their opposition to increasing salaries gave bite to a collective interpretation: that these directors were out of sympathy with and lacked understanding of college designs. The subsequent organisational change shifted considerable authority to the new board of studies and the expulsions followed. As Rayner explained it, actions were devised by the party leader in order to strengthen his power. But leadership intentions are not necessarily to be inferred from outcomes. Here, the appropriate course of action was established by the principal's calculation of *group* purposes. He identified elements — first the non-teaching directors, then the four lecturers — by their impeding the progress of the movement. However uncomfortably, the principal's outsider classifications were endorsed by the teachers who supported the establishment of and eventually became members of the board of studies. The principal's administrative authority was enhanced — within the collegiate arrangement of the board — but that was his purpose only in the obvious sense that he sought and obtained his way. That he identified a plot and sought the exclusion of its perpetrators says a great deal more about the situation of the college at that time than it does about events being directed by the principal in order to enhance his control.

The entity of the college had taken over and its purposes transcended old friendships. As with the Trotskyists, the institution of a formal structure was incompatible with the shared egalitarian view. Something had been lost — board members were not quite sure how it had come about. Was it due to an increase in workload and complexity? Or to newcomers not sharing a commitment to their idea of Chinese medicine? With regret, they accepted that more formality was required if group ends were to be accomplished. Like the principal, they harked back to the good old days when all of them fought for the just cause together. Just after the painful directors' meeting where the new board of studies had been rammed through, one of the insiders said to me:

> I just hate that sort of thing. When we all started, we were the best of mates. There was a lot of good-will and it didn't take up that much time. As the years passed we were getting more and more work and not getting anything for it. I think you start resenting that. It's a funny thing: we started off as Taoists and now the college has so many rules! I guess it's the students trying to put one over on you that gets the rules, but it's not very Taoist.

When Machiavelli and Hobbes used medical metaphors to discuss statecraft, they drew attention to the importance of cutting off serious disease early when it was relatively easy to control (in Sontag, 1983, 80-83). By comparison, Lord Shaftesbury maintained that measures designed to absolutely allay a disease 'might, instead of making a cure, bid fair perhaps to raise a plague, and turn a spring-ague or an autumn surfeit into an epidemical malignant fever'. They were ill physicians of the body politic who 'under the specious pretense of healing this itch of superstition and saving souls from the contagion of enthusiasm, should set all nature in an uproar, and turn a few innocent carbuncles into an inflammation and mortal gangrene' (in Sontag, 1983, 83). The principal had called for early attention in his own medical metaphor but purging was a treatment that might take over from the disease.

Notes

(All documents are from Australian Acupuncture College files).

1. The proposal, dated 19 September 1989, was signed by the principal, the dean of students and two co-ordinators, one of whom chaired the board of directors.
2. 'Proposal Re: Academic Staff Remuneration', 19 September 1989.
3. 'College Structure', (c. May 1989).
4. Watson, K (signed by Ferigno, P), letter to staff, 25 October 1989.
5. Giles, G. (the college administrator, writing on behalf of Watson), 21 December 1989.

VII

SHIFTING IN WITH PHYSIOTHERAPY

We fight well when we have to — we put off fighting with each other and become very united. Later, we can go back to our other disputes.

(Dean of the chiropractic and osteopathy school, Phillip Institute of Technology.)

INTRODUCTION

Chiropractors worked long and hard to get recognition. After the two disputing Victorian chiropractic associations amalgamated and secured joint participation in registration, they succeeded in getting the course located at the Phillip Institute of Technology rather than at the competing Lincoln Institute of Health Sciences which offered most of the therapy programmes in Victoria (in such areas as physiotherapy, occupational therapy and speech therapy). Lincoln teachers might have been concerned to forge the independence of their disciplines but in the chiropractic estimation their institution stood for the Australian Medical Association which was 'intent upon forcing chiropractic into a para-medical role, strictly under the control of organised medicine and physiotherapy'.[1]

The antagonism of physiotherapists counted against Lincoln getting the course. A justification given for preferring Phillip was that chiropractic would have room there for academic development and so would come eventually to be accepted.[2] The result was other: partitioning chiropractic (and then osteopathy) education from the rest — the university medical schools and Lincoln's therapy schools — only sustained estrangements.

This chapter starts with a summary of inter-occupational contentions and proceeds to the chiropractic and osteopathy school debate about joining physiotherapy in the one university.

KNOWING THE ENEMY

The Australian Physiotherapy Association (APA) vigorously resisted chiropractic recognition. It told a Victorian parliamentary inquiry on the subject (Ward, 1975) that any form of chiropractic registration, limited licensure or exemption from penal sections of the Masseurs Act (under which physiotherapists were licensed) would not only be undesirable but also would be 'detrimental to the health of the community'. While recognising the need for manipulation as part of treatment, the association maintained that 'this is best catered for by graduate physiotherapists or doctors of medicine trained in the skills and the scientific method required for complete understanding of this aspect of treatment'.[3] The federal inquiry was similarly advised. The APA argued that after allowing time for current practitioners of chiropractic to qualify in medicine or physiotherapy, 'no further person should be permitted to practise for gain as a chiropractor' (in Webb, 1977, 239).

Internal reforms were demanded to meet the chiropractic enemy without. That manipulation was a worthwhile activity now went without question. The need for greater engagement in it was frankly related to the competition from chiropractors — the 'threat' they posed. At the same time, the conviction was that physiotherapists were educationally and scientifically reputable and that chiropractors were not (osteopaths being in an ambiguous category). Physiotherapy interests and its higher healing purposes went together.

Just before the implementation of the Webb committee's recommendations on chiropractic education and registration, Maitland, the doyen of Australian physiotherapy manipulators, asked the Australian Physiotherapy Association (APA) to formally establish manipulative therapy as a physiotherapy specialty.[4] Maitland said the establishment of a specialist qualification was 'a vitally urgent one because of Chiropractic'. The urgency, he elaborated, lay in the comparison of chiropractors and physiotherapists using manipulative therapy:

> The cry made by some influential respectable members of the public, and obviously supported by chiropractors, is that chiropractors spend four or more years learning spinal manipulation; how can physiotherapists (three or more years training) with a further three months or twelve months formal

training in manipulation, hope to have the same degree of competence?

He answered that a well-trained physiotherapist who was also well trained in manipulative therapy at the undergraduate and postgraduate levels 'AND WHO HAS CONTINUED TO GROW with further clinical experience is FAR superior to ANY chiropractor'. The point was to set the training in place, and the formal qualification — he was suggesting a fellowship award to be administered by the Australian College of Physiotherapists — without delay. He believed the end result would be in the interests of the profession's patients.

Physiotherapists were at a competitive disadvantage when it came to patients. The APA's ethical code forbade professional action without referral from a dentist or registered medical practitioner. A physiotherapy educator (Galley, 1976) advocated the removal of this limitation so that physiotherapists could, if they chose, become practitioners of first contact. She began her argument by quoting the reply of a chiropractor who had been asked on a radio programme to explain the role of the physiotherapist:

> The physiotherapist is basically a second string practitioner. He is not a first contact practitioner; he doesn't directly contact the patient; he must go through the medical profession; and we feel that the physiotherapist could be used in a similar fashion by the chiropractor to provide massage and passive mobilisation of the patient (Rutledge, in Galley, 1976, 117).

This episode, Galley said, emphasised the urgency of coming to a decision about referral.

Nothing could better have secured the case for change than demonstrating that physiotherapists were publicly diminished by a chiropractor because they were not primary contact practitioners. Galley also tapped the same conceptions of occupational duties and qualities that were to be called up later in support of physiotherapy rights to acupuncture: once having opted for alternative medicine 'a patient is removed from the influence of traditional [i.e. orthodox] medicine and all the benefits it offers, including physiotherapy'; alternative medicine made much of its natural treatment approach but physiotherapy — derived from the Greek *physis*, meaning nature — also offered natural treatment within the framework of traditional medicine 'in that surgery or the prescription of drugs is not undertaken by its practitioners'. The APA removed the referral provision later that year (1976).

When the dust settled on the conflict over chiropractic and osteopathy registration, Australian physiotherapists had established themselves as primary contact practitioners and had adopted manipulative therapy. Chiropractic was used as an admonitory foil to convince physiotherapists that these changes were desirable. Nevertheless, physiotherapists were divided about the future of their occupation, an issue that turned on the established medical relation. They were as enfolded in their circumstance and as intent on finding a rightful place as were chiropractors. They wanted to get out while keeping up the advantages that came with being insiders.

Chiropractors wanted to get in while keeping up the virtues associated with being outsiders. They had no doubt about the danger posed by physiotherapy. All Phillip schools prepared what were called SWOT documents (Strengths, Weaknesses, Opportunities, Threats) for a 1988 conference run by the Institute's council. Under 'Threats' the chiropractic and osteopathy school included the following:

From a Professional Group:

The recent movement of physiotherapists into manipulative therapy is the single greatest threat to chiropractic and osteopathy because physiotherapists are:

— more numerous;
— better integrated into the public health care system;
— integrated in hospitals;
— potentially have better access to research.[5]

Chiropractors used physiotherapy as they were used by it. Like physiotherapists, they established their direction by construing enemy methods and purposes. A practitioner who had an active part in earlier struggles said about the 'traditional opposition' of physiotherapists 'Can we forget the past? Ancient history? Well perhaps 14 years ago may seem like ancient history to some — but in terms of our battle for recognition of chiropractic "It is just yesterday!".'[6] Several years later, he said:

No, I do not think I am paranoid in thinking that there are forces out there waiting to get us. The AMA and the APA may at times be prepared to sit down and talk to us, but I am convinced that it is only when they consider it to be unavoidable, and then only to use whatever strengths we might have to support their cause. Now that doesn't mean we don't try to communicate for the good of our patients, and to be honest, for the good of our profession. Quite frankly, what is good for our patients is inevitably good for the profession.[7]

The pleasure chiropractors took in making gains at the expense of physiotherapists demonstrated more than hard competition between them. Chiropractors were still the underdogs and they resented it. Their actions were often justified by references to their denigration by physiotherapists. Counter-measures were intended to even up physiotherapy advantages. National Back Care Day was a case in point. Having arranged and financed it, the physiotherapists complained that chiropractors had jumped on the bandwagon.[8] But the chiropractors were delighted to have scored at the expense of physiotherapy. When he gave chiropractic students a lunch-time talk on starting and building up a new practice, a recent graduate of the school described the strategy:

Another thing is physios organised Back Care Day. Well, chiros took advantage of it and good luck to them too! The back care thing worked well for us. We organised a shopping plaza display with free postural check-ups. Out of the 300 we checked out, about 60 of them came in and became patients of our clinics — about 85% of them had never been to a chiro or physio before.

A final year student told me of watching an interview with a physiotherapist about National Back Care Day on a popular morning-television programme:

At the end of the interview [the presenter] says — 'Then the message is: go to a specialist, your chiropractor or physiotherapist'. I was jumping around the room with excitement! He added 'chiropractor' *and* he said it first!

REPUDIATING AN ASSOCIATION WITH CHIROPRACTIC

At first, Lincoln physiotherapists and the APA went along with the idea that Lincoln should become part of La Trobe University. Then their attitude changed: the medical school at the nearby University of Melbourne offered to take over the physiotherapy course and a merger between La Trobe and Phillip seemed increasingly likely. The attraction of a medical identity and the repulsion of chiropractic propinquity joined physiotherapists in a bitter fight against the transfer of their course to La Trobe. (For an analysis of this dispute, see O'Neill, 1989.)

In its submission to a government committee (set up to arbitrate the location question), the Victorian branch of the APA opposed any training of physiotherapists in association with chiropractors and osteopaths or even having them maintained separately in the one institution: 'The comparison of qualifications consequent to the programmes being offered in the same university is unacceptable'.[9] While he made clear that he was acting in a private capacity, the president of the Victorian branch of the ACA had written to this committee suggesting that physiotherapy be shifted to Phillip where it could utilise the basic science courses taught in the chiropractic and osteopathy school and 'in effect upgrade the School of Physiotherapy from a 3 062 hour course to a 5 640 hour course . . . and also site the three professions that deal with musculo-skeletal medicine (Chiropractic/Osteopathy/Physiotherapy) together'.[10] To the physiotherapists, who came by a copy of the submission, such proposals were as abhorrent and as contrary to their objectives as the scheme for the joint conduct of manipulative therapy had been for chiropractors when they were battling years before to keep their own course away from physiotherapy.

As their dispute with the state government and with La Trobe intensified, physiotherapists continued to use the likelihood of a chiropractic presence in La Trobe as an argument against their having any connection with the university. Their status would be defiled by association. The government committee on physiotherapy location reported:

> According to the APA the [Lincoln] amalgamation agreement with La Trobe University not only threatened the close link with a medical school which supported this medical service status of physiotherapy but also opened up the possibility of affiliation with 'alternative' health science practices such as chiropractic, osteopathy and acupuncture — a situation that might lessen the professional standing of physiotherapy in the eyes of the APA.[11]

The committee was split down the middle. While the state government came out in favour of La Trobe, physiotherapists continued to fight for the medical school. A year later, an uneasy compromise was reached which left physiotherapy where it was but promised revised funding arrangements and a greater degree of autonomy for physiotherapy within La Trobe. The agreement soon broke down. The APA's Victorian branch president told a rally of staff, students and their parents that three hundred members of the association had voted unanimously to have the school moved to the University of Melbourne:

> Over and above the failure of the agreement is [the federal education minister's] publicly stated support for a Phillip Institute of Technology/La Trobe amalgamation. As you no doubt know, chiropractic is at Phillip and that would put physiotherapy and chiropractic together in the one institution. As you no doubt know, chiropractic is founded on the basic dogma that it is possible to influence and cure systemic diseases by manipulation of the spine. This is totally anathema to physiotherapists who will not wear it [i.e. any connection with chiropractic].

The APA obtained support from the medical associations. Chiropractic was portrayed in just that disreputable outcaste position from which it had sought to remove itself through improved education and registration. When the chairman of the Victorian branch of the Orthopaedic Surgeons' Association wrote to express 'our concern and outrage' about locating physiotherapy in La Trobe, he told Walker, the state minister for post-secondary education that:

> As an architect you would appreciate the importance of having a properly run professional body. The association of Physiotherapists with Chiropractors at the La Trobe University is a little bit like associating the Architectural Profession with the Builders Labourers.[12]

The letter (displayed on the physiotherapy notice board) had powerful import. In addition to distancing lowly chiropractors from an august profession, they were associated with a trade union which the Labor government had execrated and prosecuted for its fierce industrial disputation, its resort to guerilla tactics and the alleged corruption of its leader. Chiropractors were renegades. They continued to be despised and isolated as social inferiors.

The Victorian branches of the Royal Australasian College of Surgeons and the Australian Medical Association also lent their support, emphasising the affinity of physiotherapy and medical education and practice. The AMA advised the deputy premier and minister for education that La Trobe 'was the wrong institution in the wrong place to cater for physiotherapists'. There was another difficulty if physiotherapy remained at La Trobe:

The merger of the university with Phillip Institute of Technology means that chiropractors and physiotherapists would take the same degree. Because these groups vary considerably in their outlook on health care and in the final direction of their training, it would be extremely misleading for the public in the future to be unable to tell which type of practitioner they are attending. The result would be an excess of advertising, adoption of spurious or unnecessary qualifications, and in fact any means open to the practitioners to distinguish themselves: all unnecessary and undesirable from the community's point of view.[13]

Some sixteen years earlier, Cyriax, the British medical manipulator and advocate of manipulative therapy education for physiotherapists, had written in the *Medical Journal of Australia* (1973, 1165) that:

The difference between chiropractors and ourselves cannot be too strongly emphasised. Doctors and physiotherapists treat the spine for spinal disorders; chiropractors' dogma enables them to treat all who visit them. Did he but know it, when a client visits a chiropractor, the burden of diagnosis rests with himself.

The opinion about chiropractic dogmatism was unalterable. A senior lecturer in the physiotherapy department was reported in the press as saying 'It would be very difficult for us to live in the same school of health sciences as a profession (chiropractors) whose dogma is that the treatment of the spine can cure systemic diseases'.[14] This comment, along with the chiropractic and osteopathy dean's subsequent remark at a chiropractic staff seminar that there was no room for dogma in the school, led a staff member to label a spare office (which happened to contain the collected works of B.J. Palmer, safely away from students) the Dogma Room. The notice said: 'The school does in fact have room for dogma . . . Unfortunately we have lost the key!'.

GETTING TOGETHER

Teachers at Phillip were set in a turmoil by the direct engagement of the state government in formulating amalgamation plans. Its minister for post-secondary education wanted provisional statements of intent within a week and firm commitments three weeks later. Suddenly amalgamation looked to be inevitable and everybody was caught up in crisis and excitement.

There were two choices. The Phillip director had discussed amalgamation possibilities with the Royal Melbourne Institute of Technology (RMIT), located in the city centre some 25 kilometres away, and the supplier of science courses to chiropractors in years gone by. La Trobe, located only 5 kilometres from the Bundoora campus of Phillip, now took a great interest in it. Future relations with physiotherapy were central to the consideration of choices by chiropractic and osteopathy teachers. Should they incline towards physiotherapy by supporting La Trobe (where physiotherapy was still located, despite the continuing battle) or should they keep up a separation by associating with RMIT? When the dean first raised the issue with the school executive committee, he spoke of the possibility of arriving at some concord with physiotherapy: 'Maybe it's too late, but it still might be possible to put to bed this dispute between chiropractic and physiotherapy'. He suggested establishing in La Trobe, in conjunction with physiotherapy, a musculo-skeletal centre of excellence (a title for officially recognised expertise groupings that attracted additional federal money).

Another member said he had the deepest reservation about getting too close to physiotherapy:

> We are aligning ourselves with orthodoxy, we are moving away from our origins, the things that kept chiropractic in the forefront. We stand to lose our identity. It would mean that people would turn from us to the natural therapies. There are a lot of people quite worried about our losing ourselves. I tend to sense even the students from time to time say that this course is too orthodox. We do have staff members here who are telling their students to send patients down to get analgesics. Students are concerned about it.

This teacher favoured 'a separate chiropractic development from manipulative therapy in physio'. He considered it would be particularly unfortunate if chiropractic turned away from its drugless tradition 'at the very time that people were turning towards that attitude'. All the differences between chiropractors were evoked by this problem of merger choice. They condensed into a division about the future of chiropractic itself. The school was back at the crossroads.

If the chiropractors had a problem of choice, Phillip Institute and La Trobe University might well have had a problem with chiropractic. When the executive next met a week later, Phillip was on the point of deciding between La Trobe and RMIT and all the Institute schools were debating their preferences. Reporting discussions with the heads of other Phillip schools, the dean told the executive:

> The problem is thought to centre around health sciences. They are a problem in that if you continue to have physiotherapy at La Trobe then you have a problem in having chiropractic at La Trobe too. And in a RMIT amalgamation there would be the oddity of having RMIT with its [Phillip] health science school out here next to La Trobe and La Trobe having *its* [Lincoln] health science school in the city next to RMIT! One way out would be to give physiotherapy and occupational therapy to Melbourne University; we merge with La Trobe and have a health science development centered on Bundoora [i.e. a relocation of the Lincoln school to the Phillip site where it would join chiropractic and osteopathy].

The chiropractic and osteopathy school had little influence over the eventual decision about amalgamation, though this was one of those occasions when it paid to have the support of the ACA. The dean said its president had told him that the profession did not favour having chiropractic in the same institution as physiotherapy. All the same, the great ambition of the school and the profession was to have the course in a university. So one opinion on the executive was that RMIT was to be preferred, but only if it were to become a university. Another was that an association with physiotherapy had to be avoided at all costs. As the principal advocate of this position said: 'We would be swallowed up, we would become too orthodox and lose our identity . . ; If it means keeping distinct from physiotherapy, our only choice is RMIT'.

The dean also seemed to favour RMIT. He said that Phillip and RMIT shared the vocational ethos of advanced education colleges and RMIT had greater repute than La Trobe:

> The view seems to be that the public is thought to consider Melbourne [university], Monash [university] and RMIT to be the status institutions, in that order, while the perception is that La Trobe is not considered to be a proper university.

While some disagreed with this assessment of La Trobe, they were all clear that university status and better funding, especially for research, were the advantages they wanted to obtain in an amalgamation. Chiropractic would also be helped by being a big fish in a small pond; as the dean put it:

Maybe RMIT is better in that regard. We could have a division of health sciences with chiropractic continuing as a school, while in La Trobe we would be a tiny department in a large health sciences school. If we have an over-reaching division and the head goes in to fight for money, then we would be better off.

At the following meeting of all school staff, the dean said that the ACA and the executive committee thought it would be best for the school to be in an institution that did not have physiotherapy. The main RMIT health science courses were in radiography and laboratory technology and these were complementary. The staff discussed the possibilities back and forth. If they went to RMIT, one said, then they should insist that it be named a university and that the word 'Technology' be removed from the title. Another disagreed: 'I see that the practical application is the in-thing and abstract or academic approaches are out the window'. But what if Phillip ended up at La Trobe? How that was answered depended on whether physiotherapy succeeded in getting out of La Trobe and into the University of Melbourne medical school. At this point the dean dropped a bombshell:

What happens if physiotherapy stays with La Trobe? May I be so bold to make a suggestion? That chiropractic and osteopathy extricates itself from Victoria and moves to Griffith where we would be welcomed with open arms.

Griffith was a university some two thousand kilometres to the north, in the state of Queensland. But the idea was not absurd. Griffith had had a tenuous connection with chiropractic from the early days. Soon after Griffith's establishment, the Queensland branch of the ACA started discussions with it about an undergraduate chiropractic course. The university appeared receptive but felt the federal government could not be asked for funds until the recently-begun Webb inquiry reached a conclusion.[15] ACA approaches to a number of universities were mentioned in passing by the committee but it and the ACA (which remained formally attached to a university course) accepted an advanced education college course as the practical solution (Webb, 1977, 143, 155).

Charlton (the Queensland chiropractor mentioned in chapter 4) revived Griffith interest in a course but this time at the Master of Science level and to promote clinical research in chiropractic. In 1986 he presented a scheme to the university.[16] The vice-chancellor was receptive: he sought external comment, which was mixed.[17] The university wavered.[18] But Charlton worked behind the scenes to get political support and to have it conveyed to the university leaders. A meeting between them and the Queensland health minister was arranged. He read from notes supporting both undergraduate and postgraduate chiropractic education at Griffith.[19] Thereafter, Griffith pursued a chiropractic research and higher degree combination. By the following year (1988) it had announced that the introduction of the Master's course was imminent.[20] The Queensland branch of the Australian Medical Association responded by calling it 'an appalling misuse of public facilities' and by arguing that funds should be used instead to support the physiotherapy department in the University of Queensland medical school.[21]

Griffith's likely engagement was of profound importance to staff of the Phillip school. Charlton was no less opposed to dogma than they were and he also advocated the need for research (Charlton, 1986; 1987). But he attacked the school and promoted the Griffith Master's course in comparison.[22] Charlton maintained the school had failed to produce a single original research paper on spine science which had been published outside the profession's own journals. He said the school could no longer be expected to meet any further needs than undergraduate education. He also opposed Australasian Council for Chiropractic Education (ACCE) fellowship awards on the ground that they followed a 'medical specialty model'.[23] The school arranged the conduct of this programme and the first three awardees were amongst its senior teachers. Charlton said he suspected fellows were 'ill-equipped to be credible in the wider scientific and clinical community'. He also alleged that one of them was facing expulsion from the Australian Spine Society for a lack of suitable scholarly activity.

Charlton's criticisms aroused strong teacher reactions at Phillip. The school held that it provided adequate postgraduate education opportunities and that such courses should be offered in conjunction with and as an extension of an undergraduate programme. The dean wrote in defence of the school and the fellowships.[24] He also advised Griffith that it would be difficult to run a clinically oriented programme 'where no clinical facilities or clinically experienced staff exist'.[25]

Charlton now had the dean and other school staff for enemies but he had strong support in the profession.[26] There was much dissaffection with the school, which had come to a head on its commencement of osteopathy teaching in 1986. The 1987 controversy about changing the school's name to include osteopathy (which was given effect in 1988) had widened an already present breach, resulting from the barriers erected by the school against 'disreputable' professional influences. Many chiropractors believed the school had gone in the wrong direction, that is, away from the profession. So far as they were concerned, Griffith was an attractive alternative to Phillip, not only for postgraduate education but also for an undergraduate course.

Staff were dumbfounded when they were told about the possibility of moving their school to Queensland. The idea came from Charlton. He had put it to the dean some months earlier. For Charlton, the transfer would buttress the advances he had made at Griffith and meet the criticism that postgraduate education in isolation from a professional school was unsustainable. The time came when the dean, enmeshed in the complexities of Phillip's choosing between La Trobe and RMIT (over which he had little control), saw advantages in the shift. If it could be pulled off, then chiropractic would gain university status, opportunities for research would be immediately opened up, and the school would join an institution that did not have medicine or physiotherapy.

Some teachers and practitioners told me they thought the Phillip school would wither away if Griffith entered the scene. A chiropractic faculty there would have the clout that went with being in a university and the school, stuck in a college of advanced education, would be on the outer. Thus, the school would secure its continued existence by joining Griffith. Charlton had his own reason for taking out insurance. His Griffith scheme was bound to be affected if the Phillip school mounted opposition to it. Each side posed a threat to the other. Once again, chiropractic antagonists became allies for their several purposes.

The interests of the school (in maintaining its superior position in chiropractic education) and of the profession (in securing a research and educational advance) also intersected. Being close to or away from physiotherapy was a further consideration. After the dean's announcement, the staff discussion went as follows:

A: We must avoid animosity, which is between the [chiropractic and physiotherapy] associations rather than between the teachers.

Dean: We are talking about provisos — if physiotherapy remains at La Trobe.

B: Physios don't want to be associated with us, but I don't object to them being in the same building.

A: We can take the moral high ground in this: we are not rejecting them — they reject us.

Dean: We can accommodate physio in a positive way, that is, by offering a conversion course with additional work to make them chiropractors.

C: The important thing is that we try to maintain our separate identity. If we merge in an institution with physio we lose some of our unorthodox character which has led to our public acceptance. Down the line the planners will see a need to amalgamate chiropractic, osteopathy and physiotherapy.

Dean: Griffith is a realistic option. The ACA view is that a university location is good for chiropractic. They are opposed to our being associated with physio. They would push for Griffith if necessary.

C: Where the identity of chiropractic cannot be maintained, I'd prefer that we extricate ourselves from the PIT structure. Because of the expressed attitude of the physiotherapists, we would be swamped in any institution with physiotherapists in there.

Dean: What are the positive points of the moral high ground? I agree with [C] that the profession would not want us associated with physiotherapy.

A: But put that in a positive light, take the moral ground.

Dean: Because the physios have made such a hoo haa, we can appease them by extricating chiropractic.

A: Can we say that in order to overcome the difficulties made for the amalgamation by physio, we will shift chiro to Griffith?

D: We could say, 'we are very happy for you physios to go to Melbourne!'

E: You are encouraging them to have the prestige and the connection with the Melbourne medical school!

But the dean was not in a strong position with Griffith. He had no certainty about events there — the university was far from decided about chiropractic — and many Phillip staff were unlikely to want to relocate. La Trobe was more favourably regarded by the following day, when the dean held a meeting with students and a further meeting with staff. According to the dean, a student 'came up with the idea that intellectual life only prospers in temperate climes!'.

As to the staff, some had not been present the previous day and a principal opponent of association with physiotherapy (C above) was absent. Explaining the outcome of the second staff meeting to me, one teacher said:

> The majority of staff were quite for La Trobe and could live with physio, but they recognised the profession was against it. So they decided to remain in favour of RMIT still, but recognising that the tide [of opinion in other Phillip schools] was turning in La Trobe's way. This would keep them clean with the profession: they would not be seen to vote for association with the physiotherapists, even if it ended up that way.

Another gave me a similar account:

> How we ended up today was a bit of a facade I suppose. I think the majority of staff are happy to work with the physios but they recognise the strength of feeling of the profession. And after the reaction of the profession to the change of name to include osteopathy, they realise the response to association with physiotherapy would be much worse. So they can't afford for that to happen. In this sense, it's a facade.

A third (who had not been present at the first meeting) said the school had reached 'a frankly political view; it shows that it's not *us* that's against it [La Trobe] but it conveys the attitude of the profession'. He believed that chiropractors and physiotherapists could learn from each other: 'We could learn about physiotherapeutic modalities and the physios could learn from us about spinal manipulation, if they wanted to, if they were prepared to accept that we are experts in that area'.

Some teachers were not averse to combined manipulative therapy training for all three occupations — the same position Lincoln had put when it started bidding for chiropractic education over fifteen years before. Now that Lincoln was part of La Trobe, that possibility re-emerged, however distantly. The dean told me he was quite prepared to live with the physiotherapists and, besides, he feared they might take biomechanics and ergonomics with them if they departed from La Trobe to a university medical school. Lincoln had teaching and research expertise in these areas in one of its service departments and an association with them would be of great value to chiropractic. The dean took a longer view: something might well emerge out of having chiropractic and physiotherapy in the same institution. By way of example, he cited what had happened with osteopathy:

> We are already getting a confluence between chiro and osteo except with techniques. At the start we had them saying 'it has to be as it is at the British School of Osteopathy'. Then, largely through the students, this has changed. You had the osteo students saying: 'the chiro students are doing this, why can't we?'. So now they ask [chiropractic teachers] to take on this and we have a confluence of nearly everything except techniques, but even that will change.

Confluence was not without its liabilities. The osteopathy fear of being overwhelmed by chiropractic mirrored a chiropractic aversion for any connection with physiotherapy.

Even as the school shifted toward agreement about being in La Trobe with physiotherapy, continued formal support for RMIT was justified by the way physiotherapists kept disparaging chiropractic. In reporting the situation to his school board (the formal decision-making body with representation from other schools and students), the dean said:

> The chiro view was it would prefer RMIT. The school was concerned about overt expressions of animosity, antipathy and antagonism on the part of physiotherapy . . . At the [Institute] academic board [when it voted for La Trobe] the unease about physio was made and recorded. I requested it.

Equally, the opposition of physiotherapists to chiropractic continued to stand as a reason why the school might be forced to go to Griffith. Asked at the school board whether a Queensland university was a feasible or practical alternative, the dean answered that Griffith was an unknown at that point: 'It depends on various factors, including physio'. When he invited comments from the members, a student representative argued: 'Instead of having a negative approach [to physiotherapy] we should have a positive approach. We should have an approach which shows that they are not as good as they think they are!' To which the dean responded 'We should show that we didn't pick a fight, that we were forced by them . . . I don't think we will get far with them if we say that we are superior to them'.

After the meeting the dean told me that he could hardly get up in the school board and say that 'we wanted to go to Griffith because physio was at La Trobe'. But as the days went by, the Griffith possibility began to fall away. The dean did not hear more from the university and considered he could not approach it without losing a negotiating advantage. The other Phillip deans with a health science interest (from the schools of applied science, nursing, and human movement and physical education) were supportive and wanted, so the dean said, 'to see physiotherapy out of the whole thing'. They had a group interest: the state government had made a decision to leave physiotherapy in La Trobe but to keep Lincoln in the city and to spend a considerable sum on housing it there. The Phillip deans wanted to see whatever money was available spent on bringing Lincoln and Phillip health sciences together on the Phillip campus at Bundoora. According to the dean of chiropractic and osteopathy, his colleagues had agreed that:

> every possible attempt should be made to stop capital development in the city. It is not in the interest of the new La Trobe and certainly not in our interest. Otherwise twenty million is spent there and in a few years it becomes part of Melbourne University!

The future of physiotherapy at La Trobe was by no means clear since the APA and teachers continued their bitter struggle to get their course into the University of Melbourne medical school. Griffith was also uncertain and far away. The major dislocation entailed in chiropractic going there could only be justified, indeed the whole scheme could only be brought off, by the combination of a certain and clearly advantageous offer from Griffith with a clear enemy to unite the school and profession.

Griffith continued to be attractive to the dean because chiropractic 'would be a relatively important fish in a small pond', whereas at La Trobe it would be 'a very small item'. As against that, the dean and other teachers reckoned school interests could be served in the shake-up accompanying a merger of health sciences in Lincoln and Phillip. The executive agreed that Pathology ought to be in the chiropractic school, 'its proper place', rather than in Phillip's school of applied science. Apparently, the dean of the Phillip human movement and physical education school maintained that pathology should be with anatomy in his bailiwick but the chiropractic and osteopathy school maintained that anatomy, too, belonged to it. As the dean said: 'Anatomy is not in biological sciences in Melbourne University, it's in the medical school'.

The head of the chiropractic and osteopathy school's own diagnostic sciences department told the dean: 'As a department we would expect to be involved in the offer of diagnostic sciences to physiotherapists and to other departments, and to acupuncture when it comes in'. The department was not just a component of the chiropractic and osteopathy school but a power in its own right with claims to diagnostic science teaching across any Lincoln and Phillip health sciences combination.

The dean told a later meeting of the executive that 'there is still a very strong move on the part of some heads of schools to see if physio can be unstitched from La Trobe'. One strong health sciences campus could then be developed in the north of Melbourne. He had kept out of it but wanted to know what the school opinion should be. Did it mean that physiotherapy should go to Melbourne University in order to remove a barrier to a single health sciences development? As the various responses show, all but one of the members had come around to thinking that *keeping* physiotherapy at La Trobe was in their interest:

E: From a chiro point of view, the *worst* thing that can happen is that physio goes to a prestigious medical school.

Dean: From a money, strategy point of view, if the physios are able to get a new school for themselves in La Trobe [i.e. upgrading their status from being a Lincoln department to being a university school in their own right] then it improves our chances of getting a new school too.

E: We stand to gain a lot by keeping the physios. They are going to demand a lot. The demands they make are going to suit us because if they [La Trobe] give it to them, they must give it to us. It might well suit us, for example, if they [the physiotherapists] demand the incorporation of service teaching staff in their school. If another school is doing it we have a case too.

C: The only problem is if the bureaucrats get their hands on it in ten to fifteen years time and try a rationalisation of chiro and physio.

E: To be in the same place [as physiotherapy] could get us into hospitals.

Dean: What would be the impact on chiro and osteo if they went? You'd lose a very vociferous group from the university who will make all sorts of claims where, if the university is even-handed, we will benefit.

F: But if we speak out for keeping physio, then they [the physiotherapists] will see that we are riding on their backs, so to speak, and they will be all the *more* keen to go.

Dean: One of the consequences of physio going to Melbourne is that they will take biomechanics with them and that's not in our interest. What are the benefits if physio is not in La Trobe? The chiro profession will be a lot happier.

E: The profession might be all the more interested in our welfare if there *are* the two groups in La Trobe!

Dean: If we want to be totally honest, not that we always want to be, it's what's best for the training programme that ought to decide our attitude. It's better to have physios in the same institution rather than in another institution where they get a research boost. Given we are there [in La Trobe] if physios get something, we can argue reasonably that we get the same. If one analyses it, it's not clear that their being with us will be a disadvantage. They are allies in getting our service teaching in place.

A distrust of the other Phillip science school deans also came out in this discussion. They were interpreted as serving their own ends when they expressed concern about physiotherapy being in the amalgamated institution because of its antagonism to chiropractic. The dean told the executive: 'There's no bloody way it could come out that the story is that physios have been nasty to chiros and that's why they can't be in. *Their* eyes [i.e. the other school heads] are on the twenty million'.

The executive agreed with the dean's proposal — that the school should not oppose the inclusion of physiotherapy in the amalgamated institution. The dean said he would discuss this outcome with the ACA president — 'To keep the faith', added the member [C] most concerned about any dilution of chiropractic integrity. The dean nailed home the arrangement by restating the conclusion he would convey to PIT:

You have no objection if I say: our school sees no objection to seeing the retention of physiotherapy but from the point of view of the professional associations, that they have very strong views and it would be wise to keep chiro and physio separate?

Kept close at hand, physiotherapy could be used to promote school ambitions and as a lever to force distributive parities. It amounted to turning disabilities into advantages in a competitive situation. But chiropractic and physiotherapy ought not to get too close. Reporting the progress of amalgamation discussions to a later meeting of the executive, the dean said:

> Our other schools think physiotherapy should be shoved in the bay or in Melbourne University. I've conveyed our view to the director [of Phillip] and the president of the ACA: keep physiotherapy in the new university but at arms length from chiropractic.

What might come of that combination of proximity and distance was unclear. The dean wanted to open negotiations with Lincoln. He said to me with a grin:

> If we really want to make sure physio goes to Melbourne then I should ring [the acting head of the Lincoln physiotherapy department] and offer to run a conversion course that only takes three years to make a physio into a chiropractor. On the other hand, If we *really* want to hold out the olive branch we could offer to do it in a year!

Instead, he contacted the dean of Lincoln to establish an affinity of interest. Though he received a letter from the Griffith vice-chancellor inviting him to act as an adviser on undergraduate education, the dean closed off that possibility (the school executive had by now rejected Griffith). The decisive moment had arrived with the calculation that location with physiotherapy could be used to the school's advantage.

The school's position was developed in another SWOT document prepared for a Phillip discussion of the La Trobe amalgamation.[27] One of the strengths of the school was that its diagnostic science department would be unique in the university and would be able to provide service teaching to physiotherapists. Another was the significant contributions staff had made to the world medical literature on the prevention of manipulative accidents: 'This forms an important area for cooperative work between chiropractic and physiotherapy'.

The school's listing of opportunities included parity with *chiropractic* competitors:

Location of the School in a University will greatly strengthen the support it already receives from professional groups who might otherwise decrease support or provide disproportionate support to Griffith and Macquarie Universities, (who are entering the chiropractic field), merely because they are Universities.[28]

In addition, the university provided the opportunity for 'Expansion into other areas of complementary medicine as these become registered professions, e.g. : natural therapies and homeopathy'.

If the school were to become part of a La Trobe health sciences faculty then it was important that 'the "status" of chiropractic and osteopathy in the new institution is *at least* on par with physiotherapy in order to avoid outside professional interference in the affairs of the University'. Even if it was preferable for equals to stay within sight of each other, they did not have to sit together:

Because of antipathy and animosity previously expressed by physiotherapy (which has moved into the area of manipulative therapy only very recently and is therefore fighting for a share of the market), it would prevent difficulties with competing professional groups if physiotherapy and chiropractic/osteopathy remain located on separate campuses as is currently anticipated. There is no desire on the part of this School, however, to see physiotherapy relocated to Melbourne University.

PATHS TO UNITY

As the dean said, chiropractors put aside their disputes when their occupation was at risk. They did so in fighting proposed alterations to Workcare, the state government's accident insurance scheme. Chiropractors, osteopaths *and* physiotherapists were to lose their right to issue continuing incapacity certificates, that is, confirmations of worker entitlements for salary compensation while scheme-financed treatment proceeded. The effect would have been to limit renewals to registered medical practitioners who (after changes some years earlier) had the sole privilege of granting initiatory certificates. Workcare patients would be less likely to attend chiropractors, some of whom dealt with large numbers of them. The dean was actively engaged in the eventually successful campaign, which included school-organised student participation in a strike and a demonstration on the steps of parliament house. Such a resistant solidarity, which turned on maintaining current benefits, might only last as long as the issue but it demonstrated a longer-term potential to regroup under the professional banner.

Factionalism also might be overcome by the promotion of a risk to the occupation as a whole (as distinct from, in the Workcare case, a disadvantage to individual members). The invocation of an external danger has rhetorical force but other considerations are more important. While the earlier merger of the antagonistic Victorian chiropractic associations had been explained to members by the need for unity in the face of a common medical enemy, leaders saw that each association presented a threat to the other and the outcome of the competition between them for a higher education course and control of the registration body was uncertain. Solidarity was consequential upon appreciations of the several *internal* risks and led to an enduring structural alteration. Securing a continuing portion of benefits by association rather than standing to lose the lot by separation was what counted.

A third form, directional solidarity, also stems from the shared recognition of an external opponent but involves an agreement about the means of using it to secure an advantage. This 'slipstreaming' occurs precisely because members of the groups concerned see themselves as vulnerable. They forge an alliance by establishing the interests of the nearest formidable competitor and then attaching to them. For example, the overseas-trained osteopaths (represented by the AOA) saw chiropractors as an antagonistic majority whose association had tried to shut them out of registration. Yet they overcame internal differences of opinion about associating with chiropractic and supported its case for a Phillip course, thereby securing one of their own. The price was co-location with its attendant risk of subsequent absorption.

The school's endorsement of an institutional association with physiotherapy was of the same form. Settling an amalgamation direction involved reading the situation and aspirations of physiotherapists and agreeing to trade on them. That had its dangers. When a group of students was discussing what would happen when chiropractic and physiotherapy were both in La Trobe, a senior student commented 'I guess we will go our way and they will go theirs but you could see it as a medical plot to get chiro in under the wing of physio so they can control us both'.

Other students favoured accord with physiotherapy and disliked the generation of antagonism. But chiropractic was distinctive and had to remain so. Echoing the physiotherapy concern about any connection with chiropractic, a fourth year student affirmed:

> I didn't come in to be a physiotherapist. Our whole history, philosophy and attitude to health care is different. It's a good thing we will be getting a university degree and that's more important than being in the same place as physios. But because the degree is from the same place it will be supposed that chiros and physios are taught similarly or have shared teaching and standards. It will promote the idea that they are really much the same.

This student believed that most others were not opposed to being in La Trobe with physiotherapy: 'The physios don't want us but students are not saying we don't want the physios'. Teachers had adopted the same position. It would be for the physiotherapists to cast the first stone.

CONCLUSION

Concerning the experience of racially based prejudice and disparagement, Allport said (1958, 138-139): 'One's reputation, whether false or true, cannot be hammered, hammered, hammered, into one's head without doing something to one's character'. As he also noted, the awareness, strain and accommodative necessity all fall more heavily and more frequently on minority group members. So it was with chiropractors and osteopaths. Some of their responses have been considered in this chapter.

The three forms of group cohesion suggested here — resistant, consequential and directional solidarity — are always entwined, not only because many disputes are current at the one time but also because there are various external dangers. The school was united in its resistance to the danger posed by Charlton and his Griffith Master's degree scheme. But the solidarity he and the dean forged depended on the insurance consequences of moving the whole chiropractic and osteopathy school to Griffith. The threat of Griffith declined as the prospect of a La Trobe-Phillip merger advanced, but physiotherapy was the overriding danger there. The school's direction was settled in agreement that this danger could be turned to advantage.

In a merger with La Trobe the school might move (albeit tentatively) towards an accommodation with physiotherapy. But this was a contentious issue and it was put aside. Instead, obtaining benefits from physiotherapy self-improvement projects was as attractive to the school as scoring off National Back Care Day had been to the profession. The Griffith possibility became irrelevant once directional solidarity had been achieved. This, too, might only last so long as there was a likelihood of gaining an advantage out of physiotherapy's dispute with La Trobe. The future location of physiotherapy was unclear and the amalgamation with La Trobe was not sealed.

In the event, physiotherapy remained in La Trobe and a second department was established in the University of Melbourne medical school. The other Victorian medical school (at Monash University) proposed to offer a qualifying coursework Master's degree in physiotherapy for science graduates. La Trobe-Phillip negotiations collapsed (with each side accusing the other of deceit). Phillip then merged with RMIT, which was declared a university. Negotiations for a chiropractic Master's degree at Griffith also collapsed.

An overlapping debate about another aspect of chiropractic and physiotherapy relations will be considered in the next chapter. Alterations to the therapeutic capital of physiotherapy, its co-optation of manipulative therapy and acupuncture, had been a thorn in the flesh of the originating occupations. Now the chiropractors and osteopaths discussed teaching physiotherapy practices and, indirectly, acupuncture.

Notes

1. Australian Chiropractors' Association, 'A Submission on Chiropractic Course Siting to the Ad Hoc Committee on Chiropractic of the Victoria Institute of Colleges', December 1978, p. 21, VPSEC archives.
2. Victoria Institute of Colleges, 'Report, Ad Hoc Committee on Chiropractic', 8 January 1979, pp. 12, 14, VIC files.
3. Australian Physiotherapy Association (Victorian Branch), 'Submission Into the Practice of Osteopathy, Chiropractic and Naturopathy', 1973, pp.12, 16, Lincoln archives.
4. Maitland, G. 'Submission to Australian Physiotherapy Association', November 1977. Lincoln archives.
5. 'Statement for Council Conference 19-21 February 1988', SCO files.
6. Australian Chiropractors' Association, Editorial, *Victorian Branch News Bulletin* 8, 6 (1987), p. 4.
7. Australian Chiropractors' Association, Editorial, *Victorian Branch News Bulletin* 10, 9, (1989), pp. 4-5.
8. 'Back Care Day Leads to Stabbing Pains', *The Age*, 12 April 1989, p. 6.
9. Australian Physiotherapy Association (Victorian Branch), 'Submission to the Review Committee on Provision of Physiotherapy Programs', February 1988, Lincoln files.
10.Evans, J. 'Submission to the Review Committee on Provision of Physiotherapy Programs', February 1988, p.2. VPSEC files.

11. 'Report of the Review Committee on Provision of Physiotherapy Programs', Victorian Post Secondary Education Commission, June 1988, p. 21, Lincoln files.
12. Davie, B. (chairman, Victorian branch, Australian Orthopaedic Association) to Walker, E. (Minister for Post-Secondary Education), 8 September 1989, Lincoln files.
13. Hastings, R. (executive director, Victorian branch, Australian Medical Association) to Kirner, J. (Deputy Premier and Minister for Education), 13 September 1989, Lincoln files.
14. 'Fresh Talks Raise Ire of Physios', *The Age*, 13 September 1989, p. 20.
15. Rutledge, M. (secretary of the ACA's Queensland branch) to Kleynhans, A., 8 September 1975, SCO archives.
16. Charlton, K. to Webb, L. R. (Griffith's vice-chancellor), 9 May 1986, GU files.
17. Webb, L. R. to nine people who had been selected in consultation with Charlton, 16 December 1986, GU files.
18. After summarising the responses, Masters, C. (the university's pro vice-chancellor (academic)) concluded that it did not seem appropriate to proceed at that time. Undated note (April 1987), GU files.
19. The meeting was held on 5 May 1987. The unsigned and undated notes were in the form of a ministerial briefing paper for it. The notes said that many denied the scientific merit of chiropractic. This was turned into an argument for supporting investigations 'under scientific rigor such as would be applied by Griffith University, especially since chiropractors are now providing a primary contact health service'. GU files.
20. Press Release, Griffith University, n.d (April 1988), GU files.
21. Press Release, AMA (Qld. branch), 20 April 1988, GU files.
22. Charlton, K., Letter to the Editor, 'Tribute to Vision: Another View', *Journal of the Australian Chiropractors' Association* 18, 1 (March 1988), pp. 36-37.
23. Emulating medical specialty colleges was the clear intention. At the time of the transfer of the course from the ICC to PIT, the dean (then ICC principal) wrote to the ACA that it was no longer appropriate for the ICC to continue its postgraduate courses. He suggested instead that it was appropriate for the school to provide the training but that final awards for such programmes should be made available through an external body: 'The model of the Royal Australasian College of Physicians seems to be a logical one to follow'. Kleynhans, A. to Sweaney, J. (the ACA president), 26 June 1981. SCO archives. Though fellowships were awarded by the ACCE to begin with, the idea was that a college would become operative and be represented on the ACCE when a sufficient number had qualified. From the start they were called Fellows of the Australasian College of Chiropractic Science (FACCS) — also reproducing the style of Australian and British medical specialist qualifications.
24. Kleynhans, A., Letter to the Editor, *Journal of the Australian Chiropractors' Association* 18, 2 (April 1988), pp. 72-74.
25. Kleynhans, A. to Masters, C., 9 September 1988, SCO files.
26. 'Exciting Developments within Griffith University', *ACA News* 15, 4 (May 1988), p. 4. The ACA's national president had earlier told Griffith that the association endorsed the proposal and thought a university was the more appropriate place to educate chiropractors. Minty, M. to Webb, L. R., 16 July 1987, GU files.
27. 'SWOT Analysis and Strategy Plan in Relation to Amalgamation with La Trobe University'. n.d. (discussed at school executive committee on 31 July 1989), SCO files.
28. Macquarie University, in Sydney, was about to incorporate the private Sydney College of Chiropractic. The college had been sponsored by the rival United Chiropractors Association. After missing out on federal government support

for undergraduate education, it had offered science graduates a two-year practice qualification diploma. On transfer to Macquarie, this programme was to become a coursework Master of Science degree. Not only would an old enemy be gaining a university award but also it would be at a 'higher' level than the Phillip bachelor's degree. There was much school upset about the development. Macquarie was said to be diminishing the quality and status of Australian master's degree awards and departing from the norm of undergraduate education for entry to professions. A fourth year chiropractic student had a clearer view about the effect on the school: 'For the public at large ours will be seen to be a vanilla degree and theirs will be a chocolate degree with nuts on top!'

VIII

PHYSIOLOGICAL THERAPEUTICS

It is important for the student to have faith, confidence and belief in the Chiropractic adjustment while at school. After graduating the student can then learn other techniques or adjunctive therapies if he feels the need to do so . . . Electrotherapy is catered for by the physiotherapists, orthetrics by the podiatrists, acupuncture by the acupuncturists, traction by the orthopaedic specialists and clinical nutrition by the dieticians in their respective Acts and is therefore not required in W.A. for Chiropractors.

(Letter to the school from the West Australian Branch, Australian Chiropractors' Association.)[1]

INTRODUCTION

When he was asked by an osteopath to give a definition of physiological therapeutics, the dean of the chiropractic and osteopathy school explained that it was the original term for physical therapy: '"Therapies Adjunctive to Manipulative Therapy", "Physiological Therapeutics", "Physical Therapy" or "Physiotherapy" — basically, it all means the same'. What it meant for the practitioners of the original true versions of chiropractic and of osteopathy was a dilution of their central activity — the use of their hands to adjust (chiropractors) or manipulate (osteopaths), unaided by machinery or other therapies. Therein lay the problem and the source of conflict over teaching physiological therapeutics in chiropractic and osteopathy courses.

The disputants sometimes talked of equipment, at other times of procedures, and at other times again of physiotherapy, referring to the equipment and procedures habitually used by physiotherapists. In the main, the issue turned on the desirability of teaching students to apply electrical devices — ultrasound, laser and interferential therapy appliances — to reduce pain and inflammation. A machine with a vibrating head (called the G5 and used to massage sore areas) was already installed in the clinics, though osteopathy students rarely used it. The difference was that the new equipment emitted body-penetrating waves. So far as the dean was concerned, the opposition to chiropractic students using these 'modalities' (as they were also called) was due to the 'ideological bullshit of some old Palmer [college] graduates playing philosophical games'.

This question of additional therapies had a long history in chiropractic and osteopathy and in the school. Electrotherapies had become popular in medical use in the early years of this century. The original chiropractic division between 'straights' and 'mixers' turned on the adoption by the latter of electrical and mechanical devices, hydrotherapy, colonic lavage, nutritive substances and other supplements to manual treatment. National College in Chicago, where the dean had taught, was an early breakaway group (1906) that began 'mixing' in 1912 (Ransom, 1985, 49), largely on the initiative of Charles Schulze who, according to Wardwell (1992: 90) 'added "physiological therapeutics" to the curriculum (before the terms "physiotherapy" and "physical therapy" had been invented!)'. One side argued that such practices did not belong to chiropractic; that in adopting them, the profession was taking on the colour of its opponents and losing sight of the qualities that made chiropractic a unique medicine. B.J. Palmer represented this view in the most pungent terms. He was not against equipment, having introduced x-rays around 1910, announced a measuring instrument, called the neurocalometer, in 1924 which was then leased to chiropractors, and later set up in his college a piece of electrical aparatus whose name, the electroencephaloneuromentimpograph, matched its complexity (B.J. Palmer, 1939). But these were intended to assist in locating the subluxation or to experimentally confirm its existence. Equipment had its place but had nothing to do with adjusting. Those on the other side held that clinicians should use all available procedures that were scientifically acceptable and consistent with their treatment approach.

Supporters considered that what they were doing was 'natural', like the adjustment itself. On Ransom's definition (1985, 50): 'Chiropractic physiological therapeutics is the diagnosis and treatment of conditions of the body utilising the natural forces of healing, i.e. air, light, heat, water and electricity'. Historical precedents were cited in justification: all but electricity had been employed by ancient healers (chiropractors habitually traced their lineage to them), and chiropractors had taken up these adjuncts so early in the piece that they belonged to the occupation rather than to 'johnny-come-latelys' like physiotherapists.

A similar conflict had wracked osteopathy in its early years, though the use of drugs was more in contention (see Gevitz, 1982). Most of the locally-educated osteopaths had learned in a 'natural remedies' setting and were not averse to the use of at least some additional procedures. Virtually all the overseas-trained practitioners had attended courses in Britain where practice was much more likely to be 'pure' (see Baer, 1987, for an explanation of the divergence of American and British osteopathy). The advocates of 'straight' osteopathy also cited ancient healing traditions (and Still's writings) in historical justification.

The dispute continued to rage overseas. In chiropractic it was associated with the original trouble about diagnosing (which allopaths did) or analysing (the proper business of chiropractic). The mistake in diagnosing, a correspondent wrote to the U.S. newspaper *Dynamic Chiropractic*, lay in naming:

> Since the dawning of time, naming a symptom or set of symptoms has never improved the condition. For too long we have been led to believe it's important to name it. I can easily come up with 20 different ways of naming a colon than is functioning out of time with need. Or another 20 ways of naming lungs that are not operating at their optimal potential. But what would it help? Nothing.[2]

So this chiropractor, who 'even flirted with the idea of selling one of my children to purchase an electro-accustim [sic] unit', then 'sold, gave away, or trashed all of my P.T. [physiological therapeutics] equipment. I still see the acute patient and there is no more satisfying feeling than to provide help and do it only with my hands'.

As with other disputes in chiropractic, the one over physiological therapeutics pitted the ancients against the moderns. The chairman of the American Chiropractic Association board of governors reflected:

> Are we still the practitioners who built a loyal, dedicated and satisfied patient because we employed the therapeutic effectiveness of 'the laying on of hands', or have we become so sophisticated in today's modern high-tech society that we are willing to let 'machines' do what the practitioner used to do? Are we becoming so close to the medical model that we have forgotten the important ingredient — i.e. 'Touch' — that created this wonderful perception of the non-allopathic healer in the minds of those who now would introduce mandated curricula to insure some humanistic skills are

present in their respective speciality? Have we become so practice management oriented that the lure of the number of patients, and the number of dollars, has put the old-fashioned values of 'caring', 'compassion' and 'humanism' on the back burner? (Sportelli, 1989, 100).

ACA AND SCHOOL CONVICTIONS

As a creation of the ACA at a time when many chiropractors still held fast to B.J.'s thinking, the school had been against physiological therapeutics. In giving evidence in 1978 before the New Zealand commission of inquiry into chiropractic, the dean (then principal of the forerunner to the school, the International College of Chiropractic) had been asked whether the students were taught to use ultrasound. He replied 'No, we don't teach them ultrasonic treatment but they will during the course of training find out what ultrasound is all about because they have to intelligently refer to the physiotherapist'.[3] The cross-examining lawyer pursued the question: what was the main modality which students were taught to apply?. The dean said the only modality was the chiropractic adjustment. Were any adjunctive therapies taught or used by the students? No, the dean said, they were not. The lawyer kept pressing: he said he was referring to physiotherapy and electro-therapy, that type of thing. The dean was adamant 'No definitely not. We do not envisage that this will in fact become a part of the curriculum at all'.

On the advent of government funding, the ACA used its financing of the student clinics as a lever to secure an agreement with Phillip. It wanted to go on exerting a degree of protective control over clinical education and did so by having a clinical board of review set up, with strong membership from the profession. The Institute was not to provide clinical instruction or facilities without board consent and the board was to establish standards and requirements for them.[4] Therefore the school was unable to introduce techniques and devices without support from representatives of the association.

This restriction posed no great difficulty in the early days. When a teacher wanted to run a two-hour introductory session on physiotherapy concepts, the school policy was restated, namely:

that physiotherapy and other short courses of this nature, would not be taught as part of the undergraduate course. It was also

AGREED THAT lecturers should make it quite clear to the students that the lectures were a presentation of concepts only and not instructions on the use of same.[5]

However, the dean referred to requests he had for postgraduate courses in physiological therapeutics 'which could include such courses as clinical nutrition, physiotherapy, athletic medicine, acupuncture, etc.'. A 'demand' from the profession was another matter but the line was held on undergraduate instruction.

The question, as always, was where to draw the line. Several years on, the staff discussed 'Mechanically Assisted Techniques' after noting that demonstrations of the G5 machine would be introduced in 1984, along with mechanical aids to manual traction:

Discussion took place on those aspects of physiological therapeutics which the staff considered should not be taught at the undergraduate level. It was felt that the line of demarcation should be as follows. The following aspects of physiological therapeutics should not be taught in the undergraduate programme, namely electrotherapy, actinotherapy [light wave treatment], acupuncture and motorised traction. However, staff had no objections to such therapies being taught at the postgraduate level by the Institute.[6]

The restrictions were evaded. There was nothing to stop clinical supervisors using ultrasound, for example, and equipment was purchased and located in clinics. The profession was alert to any straying from the path but the school resorted to 'third party' explanations (a favourite device to get around difficulties). The dean and the supervisor of clinics told the clinical board of review that ultrasound had been introduced because Workcare (the government accident compensation authority) stated that a patient with a shoulder problem could be helped with ultrasound and the patient refused to be referred to a physiotherapist. An occupational therapist from Workcare had then said that the chiropractor in the clinic should give the patient the ultrasound required. An ACA representative recapitulated this explanation in a letter to the dean (who chaired the board) and went on to complain:

It was also stated by [the supervisor of clinics] that the ultrasound unit was only used by chiropractors who had the necessary training to use this modality, and that the unit was locked away after its use so students would not see or use it.

The statement that the ultrasound was locked in a cupboard so students could not use it or see it is surely noble, but by doing this a 'Pandora's Box' situation is being created.

Students, in their search for the magical and instant cure will surely be breaking their necks to use this 'special' off-limits modality.[7]

The next year, this member tried to get the board to agree that staff should be restricted to clinic rules (i.e. those applicable to students) but lost. Instead, the board agreed that the restrictions should be applicable to staff only insofar as they were providing care to patients who were assigned to students (meaning that students were not allowed to use adjunctive modalities on their patients and staff could not come in and do so instead). But staff, who had some of their own patients in the clinics, were not precluded 'from exercising their own scope of practice consistent with the scope as outlined in relevant Acts'.[8] The Victorian Act did not confine practice or specify allowable techniques. Thus, the leadership had succeeded in converting the absence of a limitation into the legislative presence of broad-scope practice rights. The school had edged a bit further forward in getting acceptance for physiological therapeutics.

INTRODUCING PHYSIOLOGICAL THERAPEUTICS

Changes to the membership of key committees opened the way to wholesale adoption of physiological therapeutics. A teacher explained to me:

[The dean] has wanted this course for a long time. In the past he has been blocked by people like [outside members of the profession sitting on school committees]. But [the dean] is a manipulator and he has never let the idea go. He has made sure he has got on people he knows support it. He cooked it up this time with [the head of the school's diagnostic sciences department].

And later:

What can you do with all the committee stacking on the clinical board of review and the course advisory committee [a body which also had a strong representation from the profession]. All the people who oppose this sort of thing have been replaced.

The dean had the numbers, at least in chiropractic. He brought to the course advisory committee a proposal for 'minor modifications' to two units taught by the school's diagnostic sciences department.[9] Fifth year students were required to undertake a research project and 70 course hours were allotted to it. The scheme was to offer electives instead — the research project or a 70-hour 'Therapies Adjunctive to Manipulative Therapy' (TAMT) unit. In addition, all students would be required to undertake 20 hours of introduction to TAMT. The arrangement involved a good deal of juggling of parts to fit within the existing course structure and hours, that is, it was not a 'major' amendment. Since the proposal came through diagnostic sciences rather than chiropractic sciences, possible opposition there was also short-circuited.

The item came up late in the agenda, another usual ploy. The dean explained that 'all courses that are part of the chiropractic mainstream have this unit [in TAMT]'. Students 'had to have a better understanding of what physiotherapists do so they can refer'. By introducing TAMT as an elective 'We can do a better job of the research project because fewer people will be doing it'. A member from the profession asked whether it would not be better to include TAMT in the course rather than have it as an elective. The dean said that it could be included. Another member agreed: 'It really brings our course into line with world requirements'. The alterations were approved.

The new elective was to be called 'Physiological Therapeutics' — 'the internationally accepted term'. Nevertheless, the course was often later referred to in school documents as 'Adjunctive Therapies'. When I asked the dean whether that basically meant electrotherapies, he said: 'Well, no, it extends beyond that and could include acupuncture but I have not told them that!'. The course provided an opening to bring into chiropractic a range of activities which were popular with competitors, particularly with registered medical practitioners and physiotherapists.

The course struck much more trouble at the osteopathy course advisory committee that was held immediately afterwards. The outside professional members were against it. The dean had a trump card: the osteopathy students saw physiological therapeutics coming into the chiropractic course and wanted it in their course. The chairman was caught in a dilemma. He was also a physiotherapist and 'able to use any equipment that comes along in future' but as a British-trained osteopath he was opposed to introducing the course.

He cited safety grounds (inexperienced use could cause severe burns) and the lack of teacher expertise.

Many preferred to see students doing research instead of being diverted to this activity. But the head of the school's osteopathy unit (who also opposed the course but was caught between student opinion and that of his profession) reported that the students were overwhelmingly in favour of the course rather than of research: 'These students are fearful of graduating without these skills while they don't see the absence of research as an impediment to their work in the field'. The student on the committee backed this up: 'Whether they use it or not, the students wish to know it'. The dean then put forward an argument on which a great deal turned:

> As far as students being aware of what physiotherapists do, there is a small unit [of study] in diagnostic sciences [to tell them about that]. The idea behind the elective is that with biophysics elsewhere in the course then what is offered is the equivalent of the electrotherapy taught [to physiotherapists] at the Lincoln School of Health Sciences.

Which meant the chiropractic and osteopathy students would be as qualified as the physiotherapists in physiological therapeutics. The professionals remained unconvinced. The head of the osteopathic sciences unit said he had consulted A.T. Still's writings:

> The majority of us practice ten finger osteopathy and I note Still said that if you take anything else into your store cupboard, some osteopathy leaves. We are very critical of physios taking postgraduate courses in spinal manipulation without the background. Are they going to be as critical of us?

A vote was tied, with all but one of the outside professional members opposing change. The dean and the head of the osteopathic sciences unit abstained. The committee was trapped and agreed to meet again. Afterwards, a staff member said: 'I don't think you can be both a physio and an osteopath. You have some that are both but they are more one thing than the other'.

There were also chiropractic teachers who opposed the introduction of physiological therapeutics. One told me he supposed:

> If you are part of tertiary education you have to be orthodox because it is orthodox but chiropractors have thrived by being unorthodox. It has been successful because people see it makes a

bloody lot of sense! It *does* make sense to see that health comes from within. I'm not happy about electrotherapy because the levels of electricity applied are way beyond the normal electrical activity of the body. It's an external intervention to the body, like pills or surgery. That's not what this great science of chiropractic is all about!

Another said: 'I get the feeling that we are going through this exercise so it can be included only to be excluded in a future trade-off with the physiotherapists'. His speculation was that chiropractors and osteopaths would give up physiological therapeutics in return for a physiotheraphy withdrawal from spinal manipulation. This was far-fetched since the dean believed that chiropractic owned physiological therapeutics, and the physiotherapists, at any rate, were not likely to abandon what had become an important part of their practice. But it was true that the dean hoped that physiotherapists eventually would recognise chiropractic expertise.

Other teachers were perturbed about losing the research project. If, as was likely, the majority of students elected for physiological therapeutics, then the aim of lifting up chiropractic and osteopathy by preparing graduates for research would suffer. Even when students were doubtful about physiological therapeutics (sharing the above teacher's opinion that it took them away from true chiropractic), they still had negative reasons for preferring it. Most of the students did not like the research project because it was difficult to find a topic and took up far more than the 70 allotted hours. As one said 'It's not clear what you are expected to do or what is acceptable — you just go to the lecturers and it's up to them — they say yes or no; if they say no then you just have to come back with something else that takes their fancy!'.

Some of the students also saw the loss. When the new electives came to the school's board of studies (its formal academic body), there was strong opposition to dropping research. A student representative told me:

I fought that issue about physiological therapeutics. We can't have research go like that, it's essential. There are no agreed and standardised, and validated ways of going about treatment of various conditions. You do one thing and others do another thing.

The result was that the school board modified the elective proposal by requiring that half the students continue to take the research project.

A REVISED PLAN

The dean reconsidered his position. He circulated a discussion paper to the school executive committee.[10] By this stage, the explanation for the introduction of physiological therapeutics had shifted to third parties. The dean wrote that the impetus for an elective had come from:

a) [the] Chiropractic Clinical Board of Review who felt that the Institute could be accused of presenting a sub-standard program in view of the absence of adjunctive therapies from the curriculum while being included in the programs of all mainstream colleges — in most cases as an integral part of the undergraduate degree course;

b) the Course Advisory Committee in Chiropractic where some members oppose the introduction of an elective in favour of integration of adjunctive therapies as a required component of the course.

The dean maintained that the fifty/fifty scheme was impossible, not least because the head of diagnostic sciences had indicated that an additional half a staff member would be required to supervise research. If physiological therapeutics were dropped, then a similar problem remained in staffing the research project. Further, the school would be letting the profession down because elements of it would regard the whole course as deficient and 'we will not be meeting the requirements of chiropractors who require training in order to allow them to utilise procedures available to them in practice by law'. His final consideration was 'If adjunctive therapies are not introduced in 1989, it may not in future be readily introduced following amalgamation because of potential opposition from physiotherapists at La Trobe University'. The dean suggested a complicated solution which allowed electives in both the student research project and physiological therapeutics (the latter to be called initially 'electrotherapy/actinotherapy/mechanotherapy') and added an epidemiological study for all students which would be based on their own cases in the student clinics.

The dean's argument at the executive committee was that students could easily fit in the additional research study: 'People can in most cases meet their [clinic patient] quotas well within the hours — they often sit around in the clinics doing nothing or watching television'. The plan was modified again, but this time in the direction of full implementation. Students would have research/

physiological therapeutics electives as part of their fourth year diagnostic sciences course in 1990. Thereafter, the research project would be discontinued and physiological therapeutics would be taken by all students. The epidemiological research component would be added to the chiropractic clinical programme, together with a requirement that one hundred applications of physiological therapeutic techniques be completed. If osteopathy students wished to qualify in physiological therapeutics then they would have to produce evidence of having completed one hundred applications in their clinical residency.[11] The significance of this last point was that supervisors in the school's osteopathy clinic were neither qualified nor interested in the use of electrotherapies. Therefore osteopathy students who wanted to complete the 'application' requirement would have to seek out osteopaths who used these procedures and gain attachments with them during the six-month internship after the school course ended.

When this arrangement was discussed by the school's board of studies, the dean gave the following reason for including physiological therapeutics as a necessary part of the course: to do otherwise complicated budget planning 'so when that was realised we gave adjunctive therapies to everyone — it makes them able to work as part of the health care team'.

A difficult argument started over the one hundred treatment requirements. Students would use the equipment just to get their numbers up; nevertheless, some minimum had to be specified to ensure the students were properly trained in the use of the equipment. 'You just can't force someone to have an ultrasound treatment if the student and the clinician feel it is not justified', said one staff member. Another backed him up: 'If you put in one hundred operations [as a requirement] then you will get one hundred but that does not mean it is justified. The implication is that our philosophy is to *encourage* the use of these modalities'. A third said: 'We need a quota but people can cheat, not to put too fine a point on it. You can give ultrasound to various places on the one patient and end up with twenty patients having one hundred applications'. A student chimed in: 'We are confining the patient to the technique, not the technique to the patient'. The dean got around that by saying the clinical board of review would monitor the quota requirement. There was a silence. Then the proposal was moved by the teacher who was most opposed to the whole scheme and seconded by another who also had doubts about aspects of it. And so it passed.

In the grumbling afterwards, teachers who had voted for the plan maintained that treatments would, to some extent, be pressed on patients to meet the quota requirement rather than matched to their conditions. If students had to do a certain number of things then they found the patients to do them on: they *made* the need. But maybe that was the aim, they said, to carry physiological therapeutics through into subsequent practice so that graduates used it – the basis for doing so having been settled by the requirement. They agreed that the certification in physiological therapeutics, as one put it, 'aint worth shit – one hundred applications, what does that mean? But the trouble is, the people who get it will *believe* it'.

For his part, the dean was unhappy about a student who had been less than generous in his support for physiological therapeutics at the board meeting: 'One of the students must have a straight background!'. A senior colleague commiserated: 'It makes it hard when you have to represent students'. This touched a common interpretation of member action at school meetings. If a view was not liked then (a) the person was not expressing a 'real' opinion but one that she or he was constrained to put as a representative; or (b) the person was pushing her/his own view and not 'really' representing group opinion; or (c) the opinion, precisely because it was representative, indicated that the assertor blindly followed group tenets (of the straights, for example).

The reverse also held. The dean could maintain that physiological therapeutics was not *his* idea. He corrected a staff member who spoke as if it was: as the dean he was representing the executive committee's proposal. Again, the head of the osteopathic sciences unit had committed himself with students not to oppose physiological therapeutics but an osteopath (who, like him, opposed the course) had told the head that his place on the course advisory committee was to represent teachers, that is, to oppose the course because they did.

Representation also stood for group loyalty. The teacher who had moved the motion explained afterwards that he had felt a moral obligation to do so, having voted for it on the executive. Why had he supported the course on the executive? He said that he had fought the introduction of physiological therapeutics for four years but now felt outnumbered. When the professional association, the ACA, began to express its concern about compulsory physiological therapeutics (arguing instead that the course should be optional), the dean told one of the ACA leaders that this teacher had moved the motion that it should be accepted as a compulsory course for students. Thus, *individual* support for an action, despite the well-known contrary views of the person concerned, could be advanced to legitimate a group decision when it faced external criticism.

BELIEF AND INTEREST

One might explain the action of the dean and others who supported the introduction of this subject by their interest in protecting and enhancing the strategic position of chiropractic. But the explanation is insufficient. Of course, they were concerned about chiropractors being left behind by phsyiotherapists; also, they were convinced of the worth of physiological therapeutics, the rightness of the use of these therapies by chiropractors, indeed their historically-evidenced prior claim to them. As the dean told me:

> Look, I know. I practised as a straight chiropractor for many years. Then I went overseas and learned these things and came back and used them in my practice and helped people with them who had not been helped as much before by straight adjusting. I know that ultrasound and the like can be very beneficial.

The scientific merit of electrotherapies was not raised in any of the debates I attended. The issue was not to be decided by a consideration of experimental evidence. Only one teacher privately questioned efficacy, citing a negative trial report and a literature review article which found no substantiation of claims for ultrasound (Williamson et al., 1986; Partridge, 1987). This teacher was opposed on the principle that electrotherapies formed no part of true practice and the papers were supplementary to his argument. Obviously, the supporters believed that electrotherapies were beneficial but this was a background understanding. The issue did not hang on the science of electrotherapies but on (a) their suitability for chiropractors and osteopaths; and (b) the consequences if they did not take them up. As with the issue of school location, strategic considerations helped to secure group accord. This became more evident in the next round of the physiological therapeutics saga.

The compulsory course plan had now to pass the chiropractic and osteopathy course advisory committees. Osteopathy was the first hurdle. The head of the osteopathic sciences unit reported the predictable opposition of course teachers. They, and the professional association, were happy enough about a postgraduate course but not about any undergraduate provision. Faithful to Still's precepts, a member of the profession spoke for all but the one who had previously voted for the course:

> We don't have enough time in five years to teach the osteopathic concept without adding courses that are irrelevant . . . Anything that allows you to not use your hands, that detracts from the principles and philosophy of osteopathy, waters down your competence as an osteopath.

Another osteopath said 'We practise manual therapy and we don't want a dilution of that; in no way do we want to be seen as competing with physios who we see as operating satisfactorily in this field'. They traversed all the old arguments. But when it came to a vote, the scheme passed. The professionals, with the same one exception, were against it while the student representative, two chiropractors (including the dean) and a medical practitioner were in favour.

The result confirmed osteopaths in the opinion that chiropractors were railroading them. At a later meeting of the executive of the AOA, the change was joined with other examples to confirm what all feared: osteopathy was being merged in chiropractic. One executive member said: 'The poor students, they are supposed to be doing an osteopathy course but no wonder they are having trouble, they are taught all the time by chiropractors!'. But the students had been in favour of the course and *they* added opposition to it from the profession to their catalogue of resentments about the AOA. Things would be different, they said, when they had graduated in sufficient number to take it over.

Explicit ACA opposition to the introduction of a compulsory subject had its effect at the following chiropractic course advisory committee. One member of the profession who had been strongly in favour previously now said that whilst his *personal* sympathies were for a required unit he was bound by the current ruling of the ACA to support electives in research and adjunctive therapies. The dean returned to the question of representation: 'They are here to speak in their own right, not to speak on behalf of their associations. They are here as persons, not as representing an outside body'.

Two members of the UCA (the other chiropractic professional association) were present and in favour of a compulsory unit. People from the group who had been most at odds with the school in earlier years supported it on this issue while those from the group who had established the forerunner of the school were opposed. The incorporation of physiological therapeutics was a congenial scheme for members of a body that had been set up to represent locally-trained practitioners using a variety of therapies. Many ACA members now thought likewise but in backing electives the association was steering a middle course between its divided elements.

The options — a compulsory unit of research and physiological therapeutics electives — were both displeasing. The teacher most opposed to the new course argued that research had to be preserved in the school but very few students would undertake it if they had the opportunity to do physiological therapeutics instead. A chiropractor (who did not support the ACA stance) responded: 'It's all about treating people, that's the profession's charter and using these modalities helps people. Only 2% will do research'.

The dean maintained that the introduction of physiological therapeutics had first been suggested to him by the head of the diagnostic sciences department as a means of coping with financial constraints. That is, an external consideration obliged the school to adopt the subject. Then there was the threat of the physiotherapists. The argument earlier had been that physiological therapeutics had to be started before the La Trobe physiotherapists had the opportunity to stop it after amalgamation. Now the case shifted to the school's exposure if physiological therapeutics were not compulsory. The dean asked:

> If physiological therapeutics is not an integral part of the course but an elective, do we see any danger in losing it if we are part of La Trobe by 1 January 1990? Do we see any difficulty in physiotherapy objecting to it in 1990?

He was backed by the ACA chiropractor who favoured a required unit: 'There are a lot in our profession, reactionary forces, who do not want physiological therapeutics in *any* form. It would suit them very well if the physiotherapists opposed!'.

This struck another responsive chord. It was near-standard practice to describe internal opponents in terms of their siding with, or leaving the profession open to, external antagonists. Their rabidity was construed by the tactics they employed rather than by their beliefs as such. They were made into enemies of the true mission by giving external enemies a purchase for subsequent exploitation. All sides to a dispute found reason to define adversaries in this manner. It would not have been so without a shared fear of submergence.

THE RESULT

As in the debate over transfer to La Trobe, the invocation of physiotherapy had a powerful effect on the outcome. During a period when I was away from the school, a required physiological therapeutics course was approved for introduction at the start of the following year. The section on laser therapy contained lectures on Chinese meridian theory, the idea being that the device should be applied to acupuncture points. The students were not being prepared to practise needle acupuncture but the presumption was that the principles of this medicine were to be absorbed. The school was moving outwards to embrace 'natural' therapies in its domain.

The prospect of an amalgamation might not have been decisive. There were other reasons for wanting a course, such as maintaining parity with overseas colleges, sustaining the claim to physiological therapeutics, acting on the conviction that patients were assisted, and (on the part of the 'service' diagnostic sciences department, which would conduct physiological therapeutics) enhancing its position in the school by teaching a clinical programme. The competitive situation was a stimulus to act before physiotherapists might be in a position to mount opposition to the school's adoption of 'their' therapies.

The dispute subsided but after the course had been introduced and electrotherapies were being used in the clinics, the original issue of chiropractic distinctiveness re-emerged. A fifth year student told me:

> This woman came into the clinic yesterday and, tentatively, I decided to give her interferon therapy. I said to her, 'Today we are going to use this machine to give you gentle relief' and she says, 'Is that the one with the suction cups? — I've had it already last week with the physiotherapist'. Right, I think, we've got to be doing something different to the physios, so I gave her an adjustment!

Another fifth year student considered that it had been useful to learn the electrotherapies. Previously, he would have referred patients to physiotherapists for this form of treatment but now, having seen how little there was in it, he realised that 'the grass is not greener on the other side' and he would be much more inclined to persevere with his own treatments. He said: 'It's an irony that we are taking over their therapies just as they are taking over ours. I don't mind [physiotherapists] doing manipulative therapy so long as they don't say at the same time that it doesn't work'.

SUMMARY

There continued to be differences about the place of physiological therapeutics in chiropractic and osteopathy but the school did not fall apart over the issue. As with the amalgamation debate, agreement was reached by projecting physiotherapy advantages onto chiropractic and osteopathy. The danger was reversed in an amalgamation: physiotherapists might stop the school from extending its activities — teaching the use of equipment and procedures that were, so some advocates like the dean thought, theirs by right. However, the opponents of adjunctive therapies did not want to save their medicines from outside influences, like physiotherapy, but from those of their own who would subvert the original and true messages of chiropractic and osteopathy. External and internal enemies were always mixed together in a reckoning. Advancing the medicine and defending earlier gains were aspects of the one cause.

As suggested earlier, a variety of considerations lead members of a group to a single position — the emphasis shifts back and forth between identifications of threat and interpretations of purpose. Their solidarity is distorted by reducing it to one or another mode of collective action directed to certain ends, as in Parkin's (1974, 1979) attempt to distinguish groups by reference to their typical exclusionary or usurpatory closure strategies. Faced with a critical issue, which may remain in the background for years as was the case with physiological therapeutics, the people involved are engaged in deciding what they stand for and what to do. Yet they do not decide in the abstract: chiropractors, osteopaths and traditional acupuncturists settled their collective actions by typifying what they understood to be the exclusionary and usurpatory pursuits of *others*, within and without. Alliances, however frail, obtained their meaning in this way.

Notes

(All documents are from the school of chiropractic and osteopathy files and archives).

1. Rose, B. (secretary, W.A. branch, ACA) to Kleynhans, A., 2 October 1986.
2. Kelly, R. Letter to the Editor, *Dynamic Chiropractic* 7, 19 (1 October 1989), p. 42.
3. New Zealand Commission of Inquiry into Chiropractic, *Transcript of Evidence*, 20 December 1978, vol. 14, p. 3 264.
4. 'Terms of Reference', Clinical Board of Review, n.d.
5. Minutes, Chiropractic Sciences Meeting, 15 September 1982.
6. Minutes, Chiropractic Sciences meeting, 8 February 1984.
7. Hinwood, J. to Kleynhans, A., 3 October 1986.
8. Minutes, Clinical Board of Review, 30 May 1987.
9. 'Minor Modification to Diagnosis and Management II and Diagnosis and Management III', n.d. (circulated for the course advisory committee meeting held on 16 May 1989).
10. 'Discussion Paper on the Introduction of an Elective Unit in Adjunctive Therapies', 29 May 1989.
11. 'Discussion Paper on Minor Modifications to the B. App. Sc. (Chiropractic) and the B. App. Sc. (Osteopathy)', 6 June 1989.

IX

GOING BY THE BOOK

A word of advice: STUDY HARD and PARTY HARD. It's all a matter of pacing yourself.

(President's message, Chiropractic Students' Association Newsletter).[1]

Why the comment that heavy hours turned the course into a lifestyle? Why that? It *is* a lifestyle, a wonderful one! This is an amazing comment.

(Chiropractic practitioner commenting on reported student concerns about workload.)

GETTING IN

The dean of the chiropractic and osteopathy school gave a welcoming speech to arriving students. He told them that the ideal of service was important:

> Both professions provide a very nice way of earning a living, of realising your goals, of caring for people and of being financially independent. Yet, because of this, your chosen discipline demands of you the dedication, commitment and sense of responsibility becoming to a professional in the health field. You will no doubt be reminded of this from time to time . . . Happiness comes from success and success is the progressive realisation of a worthy ideal.

New acupuncture students were also told of their duties but their task was different. Instead of having to line up to standards that were already set, they had to help make their occupation into a profession. During their orientation, a speaker explained that 'professions develop to exclude those who are sub-standard — this is why professions develop to make it exclusive, and sometimes expensive'. The college principal followed on:

We will do all we can to make you capable and competent. We will not let you out unless you are competent. You have to get yourself known. It's absolutely essential you promote the profession. Some of them out there are absolute charlatans.

The acupuncture college and the chiropractic and osteopathy school had this in common: graduates were to demonstrate moral as well as technical qualities. Like unruly Nature, the students had to be shaped and ordered to their professional ends. That dour endeavour began with their admission.

Chiropractic and osteopathy programmes attracted far more applicants than there were places available, which drove up entry requirements. Then the fact that successful applicants had to obtain high aggregate examination scores was held to evidence the quality of the school. That demand exceeded the availability of student places 'by several hundred percent' was reported as a strength of the school in one of its 'SWOT' documents.[2]

All candidates were interviewed. Some teachers questioned whether academic success could be predicted in this way (e.g. Lines, 1989 c) but interviews were directed to establishing whether applicants had 'an enthusiasm for the practice of healing, a willingness to explore new concepts in health care, good mental and physical coordination and a high level of integrity'.[3] Members of interview panels — they were drawn from practitioners, senior students and teachers — were to advise on the applicants' commitment to healing, understanding of the nature of chiropractic or osteopathy, social responsibility and motivation 'to undertake an arduous five year course of study'.[4] That was a tall order for a 15 to 20 minute interview.

Usually there were three members to a panel and each completed a tally-sheet for each candidate.[5] They were to be rated on attitude, appearance, self-assurance, maturity, sense of purpose and so on. The whole procedure culminated in a panel ranking, from being strongly-for to being strongly-against admission. In most instances, aggregate examination marks rather than interview results determined eventual selection of those who were applying straight after leaving school. A high interview recommendation would only compensate for a low aggregate mark in unusual circumstances. Conversely, an applicant with an examination score well above the likely minimal level for entry but with a low interview recommendation was likely to be admitted.

Many of the practitioner and student interviewers (and some of the staff) did not know how selection was worked out following their involvement. The interviews counted for them, as they did for the applicants, because they were assumed to be vital to the outcome. Even if interviews were of questionable worth as a device for picking candidates likely to succeed in the course or in the profession, they gave expression to the personal qualities that teachers and practitioners considered important. The interviews also had the great advantage of drawing practitioners back to the school. Those who were invited to be on the panels were helping the school, their school.

Candidates were also interviewed because of school concerns about doctrinaire and mercenary tendencies in the profession. As a senior visitor to the school put it, their purpose was 'to sort out the kooks and those interested in it for the money'. That might amount to the same thing, since cultists were often accused of being money-grubbers. The school was as concerned to keep out the wrong sort as it was to find the right sort to admit. Though the aim was to discover candidate attitudes during interviews, panelists settled on *their* opinion about each of the candidates. In doing so, they consolidated understandings of their own professional worth. The annual interview cycle took on ritual significance as an affirmatory occasion. Occupational and personal virtues were refracted through the passage of applicants.

A stimulus for this solidary exercise was provided by items on the check-list. For example, panels were to rate the dress of candidates on a scale from 'exceptionally neat and tidy' to 'positively untidy'.[6] Dress showed how much applicants cared — how important it was for them to get into the course. As a senior teacher explained to me: 'If they don't have the wit to dress well for an interview, what will they have the wit for?'. Besides, if chiropractic and osteopathy were true professions, as all believed, then practitioners would confirm it by dressing as professionals did. Imaging the surface characteristics of respectability was not so much contrived to evidence worth as it was intuited as a response to disparagement. The seemliness of attire dispelled any whiff of quackery. Later, students would have to dress the part in clinics. Looking too feminine could be a problem. As a female student said: 'Even though you are dressed up, you are let know it would be more appropriate to have grey pants and a nice ironed blouse'.

A group of fourth year students discussed interview panels, on which they had recently served, during an evening meal. They agreed that interviews were needed. It made sense not to choose just on marks : 'After all, with one exception that's what the medical schools do [i.e. not interview applicants] — and you get people going into medicine with no understanding of its human part'. Another said: 'Sometimes they [the applicants] were so close, there was nothing we could make a distinction on but dress'.

In summary, interviews were an annual renewal of the school's occupational improvement project and an initiation for its students. Panel recommendations were acts of confirmation: it was not so much that selectors agreed about the applicants to be chosen as that interviews were an occasion for the ratification of occupational worth — what chiropractors and osteopaths were supposed to evidence in their practice rather than what, in many instances, they did evidence. As the dean made clear in his welcoming speech, new students were select people and the financial rewards established the duties of their high office as professional healers.

Acupuncture teachers were no less concerned that applicants possessed the right intentions. However, they wanted to fill enough places to keep the college going financially until it entered the university. This imperative was not in conflict with the appraisal of candidates for they were considered to be self-selecting. Like chiropractic and osteopathy students in earlier years, the act of seeking out an 'irregular' course and being prepared to pay for enrolment in it was held to demonstrate a worthy interest.

The prior education and experience of candidates would have sufficed to get most of them into official tertiary courses. During the period from 1986 to 1990 inclusive, 34% of those entering the acupuncture programme were employed and/or qualified in health occupational fields; 12% had enrolled straight from school; 9% were teachers; and the remaining 45% had a great variety of work and previous education (over half of them at tertiary level). On average, they were 29.5 years old on admission.[7]

Each applicant was asked to write an essay giving reasons for wishing to study acupuncture. Nearly all saw it as a possible end to their searching for a fitting combination of life-mission and occupational engagement. The following is representative: 'I would like to study acupuncture because I want to earn a livelihood in a way which is compatible with my view of the world'. Another essay commenced:

> To explain my reasons for wishing to study acupuncture, I should, I suppose, include my whole life story and how I arrived at this point at this time, like a thousand tributaries running into a river before it flows into the sea, but with only two pages available I will try to be brief.

Candidates identified acupuncture with holistic and natural approaches to healing, the Chinese philosophical integration of mind and body and the harmonisation of energies. Acupuncture was an alternative, not completely perhaps, but a personally and socially redemptive one. An applicant wrote of his growing realisation, demonstrated by experience in health promotion, of 'the inability of the traditional western medical model to adequately explain and, in many cases, treat the causes of ill-health'. Another explained: 'It is the wholistic approach of acupuncture which fascinates me, and in terms of alternative therapies it is such a traditional form of treatment, virtually the Grandfather of alternative therapy'.

The insufficiency and damaging consequences of much orthodox treatment were often cited as reasons for turning away from regular medicine. One, who was for drug-free therapy, wrote: 'Without wishing to deride the marvellous surgical techniques and equipment available to modern medicine, I still think a lot of common medical problems are treated with the "mask the symptoms but don't find the cause of the problem" mentality'. A nurse said that after regularly getting feedback from patients about their various medications and the side-effects they encountered, she was prompted to look for other modes of treatment, especially for pain control, anxiety and stress. Another nurse wrote: 'My belief is that western medicine is superficial – a case of visiting a doctor and receiving a prescription'. And another said: 'What fascinates me most is that in today's life, when many people are aware of the urgent need to come back to nature and help not only heal it, but themselves, Traditional Chinese Medicine seems to be just at "the right place, in the right time"'.

For all their differences in age, employment and education these students commenced with an affinity for and sometimes a fair knowledge of acupuncture. Whether it was acceptable in western scientific terms was far less important for them, and for teachers, than Chinese metaphysical thought and its medical application.

Acupuncture was a bond and at the beginning of each of the two years I was there, opposition to the NH&MRC was the rallying call.

ACCESS, EQUITY

Like all the other higher education institutions, Phillip espoused equal opportunity in the admission of students. That got down to knotty problems of balancing the sex composition of the intake and of securing places for those who could show disadvantage. The Institute had a policy on these matters but whatever the issue, Institute policies were likely to be regarded as impositions and as threatening a small and vulnerable school. Thus, staff did not oppose the principles of equity and access; they did, however, treat any Institute promulgation with suspicion.

An Institute report on equity targets and progress towards their attainment came to the school executive committee.[8] It met with immediate resistance. 'For one thing', the dean said, 'half our students aren't female'. A senior teacher (a woman) responded: 'We'll make half of our students female when nursing makes half of its students male!'. 'I couldn't say it better', the dean replied. He drew attention to another Phillip document singling out courses with less than a 45% female enrolment (34% of the chiropractic students were women).[9] 'Absolutely ridiculous!', the previously quoted teacher said. But some response had to be made, and the executive agreed to set enrolment objectives of 35% females for the chiropractic course and 40% for osteopathy — in the knowledge that these levels had already been reached or exceeded over recent years.[10] A performance which was more incidental than intentional proved that the school had taken the Institute's policy to heart and was keeping up with it. The defensive stance settled the response. That went for the professional associations too: really, it was *their* problem. The dean suggested writing to them, since, as he said, 'there couldn't be more than 10% females in chiropractic'. (Between 1979-1989, the school graduated 547 chiropractors, 18.8% of them (103) being women).[11]

The executive turned to another heading in the Institute paper — Aborigines. The earlier-quoted senior teacher commented: 'There's a strong argument for them, provided they meet academic requirements. Mind you, they would not go back and work with Aborigines'. 'That does not count!', the dean replied. Next were disabled persons. 'Only disabled persons who are capable of doing the job!', this teacher said. Another senior teacher added: 'Anything there yet about lesbians and homosexuals? Surely *they* will be the next to come up! I'm only being ridiculous, but goodness gracious!'. Next was child care. 'They say we have to provide child care!', the dean said. The female teacher was rather in support of that: 'I don't like having children in my classes!'. Then there were opportunities for people who had left school before completing a full secondary education. The executive agreed they might be considered, provided they had done the normal bridging courses. The dean concluded the item, saying: 'Anything else we can do about equity? Chiropractors and osteopaths are minority groups. Is there anything we can do for them? Put it down!'

To repeat, individual teachers supported policies directed to assisting the entry of disadvantaged applicants but their *collective* resistance was influenced by the source of the equal opportunities paper. When the school registrar raised the issue of female participation with the executive, her firm demands for action were respected and, within the overriding limits set by the quality argument, accepted. (She was absent on this occasion.) When those defined as outsiders raised the same issue, the group did not take any action it had not already taken. It had not, as the Institute policy required, made a plan to improve matters.

Apart from the head of the diagnostic sciences department, the chiropractic course teaching staff were male, with several female supervisors in clinic out-stations. One of the clinics was preferred by some women because of female supervision. Some male chiropractic students typed osteopathy as a female course and, by association, as a soft option. This was most likely to occur where students had taken up the hereditary antagonism to osteopathy and opposed its co-location. The osteopaths were reduced to masseurs and that went along with their being female.

There was a strand of rough masculinity in chiropractic. The jokes brought it out. The following 'advertisement' appeared in an early edition of a resurrected student newsletter:

Figure 7   Extract from student newsletter

NEVER BE ALONE AGAIN

If you're tired of chasing her all over the farm and then find she's not in the mood

THE INFLATABLE SHEEP

Proudly made in
NEW ZEALAND

FEATURES:

Kissable lips, Bleating
sounds from the latest
Digital electronics (Use
the plug in your
Walkman's headphones
(specially suitable for
flat dwellers)

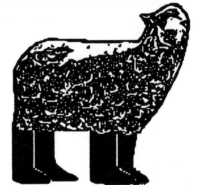

Edge of cliff function so that she pushes back that bit harder.

Supplied with a free set of Gumboots (specify size) and
lanol spray for the authentic shearing shed smell.

Run on 240 volt or batteries.

YOUR FANTASIES CAN COME TRUE

(*The Axis*, vol. 2, 30 April 1990).

A gossip column had these items:

Did any one notice the love bite Matt Seisun had on his neck early last week? It was a real ripper and very hard to hide — as Matt found out (the collar wasn't quite big enough was it Matty?). Anyway have a good look at his neck there may still be some remnants left!

Certain blonde Echuca 4th year female was seen forcing herself upon innocent and totally 'unwilling'? 3rd year male (of the initials — P.D.). Did he discover the contraindications of succumbing to the attentions of a very drunk and slightly nauseous blonde.

Mr. Jag Man of 3rd year seen leaping into bed with two innocent chiro girlies, dressed in his bow-tie and a pair of boxer shorts.

The Phillip students' association took exception:

The Student Union will not support any publication in which women are portrayed as objects of men's sexual and/or violent fantasies. I have had reports from a number of people who found much of your newsletter not only deeply offensive, but bereft of any useful information regarding your School, a view I have to agree with.[12]

This tapped the familiar chiropractic interpretation of attacks. The editor commented in the next edition:

It seems that when anyone embarks on [a] new project they are often the subject of criticism.

As a result of this letter I surveyed the women chiropractic students in order to gain a perspective in answers to many of their criticisms. I received a disappointing 37% return of questionnaires (maybe this reflects these issues importance to women students) . . . I apologise if we have offended anyone as this is not our intention. Some of the responses and comments I received are diametrically opposite, highlighting the old adage that you can't please all of the people all of the time.[13]

Of the respondents, 8% had been offended by items in the newsletter; 14% thought the newsletter perpetrated sexist and/or derogatory attitudes; and 9% agreed that women were portrayed in it as objects of men's sexual desires.

Given the size of the female enrollment and the limited response, the percentages did not indicate much.[14] Women were a minority within a group that was sensitive to its minority position but that did not lead to a particular sensitivity to women. They frequently referred to unsatisfactory male attitudes and presumptions.

The acupuncture college had a similar sex distribution: 32% of the 1986-1990 college entrants were female. Most teachers and all the leaders were male. Since classes only came together on Sundays and one or two evenings a week, students were not in such frequent contact with each other as were the chiropractic and osteopathy school students. Males sometimes dominated class conversations in the early years but the atmosphere was less inimical to women. They occasionally spoke critically of individual male teacher behaviour but scarcely ever (at least in my hearing) of male students.

KEEPING UP REPUTABILITY

Patients might recognise the worth of chiropractic, osteopathy and traditional acupuncture but associations representing registered medical practitioners and physiotherapists obviously did not. That had its effect on students. 'The trouble is, it rubs off onto you', a fourth year student said, referring to disparaging remarks in a medical journal article. 'You end up being niggard about the medicos'.

Writing about the New York chiropractic students he studied, Sternberg (1969, 236) explained that his purpose was:

> to convey to the reader the picture of chiropractic students surrounded or besieged by hostile groups and forces . . . The image then is of a threatened self — torn between its own relatively positive and worthwhile view of the status of chiropractic student and the negative view of most of society. The self is torn because . . . it is so intensely aware of the 'bad' evaluation of chiropractic, chiropractors and chiropractic students made by most people.

Phillip students reported experiences of antagonism and prejudice about their choice of occupation but scarcely ever from relatives, friends or casual acquaintances. 'It's just one of those things that happens', a teacher (and school graduate) said:

> At social gatherings, for example, mainly from physios and doctors and even more so from the people they are married to — actually, they are the worst! Their minds are fixed from received information. With ordinary people it does not happen at all. They are quite interested in your being a chiropractor.

Students were made indignant and uneasy by continued denigrations of occupational worth. That could become apparent in relations between them. A fourth year student told me of being treated as a pariah by his class. He was outspokenly critical of teaching quality and teacher attitudes, comparing both unfavourably with his university experience: 'The way some of the staff like [a named teacher] lord it over you, and some of them are not qualified!'. If one complained too much and in the wrong way then a line was crossed and the critic joined the enemy. Another student had said to him: 'Why don't you f . . . off and do medicine?'.

On the one hand, students were told that their future occupations had attained recognition, that they were being prepared to enter the health occupational mainstream. On the other, they participated in teacher and practitioner representations of the insufficiencies and dangers of orthodox practice. The chiropractic science department had a policy that:

> no other health care groups should be denigrated in the teaching or discussion of principles, philosophy or in general as it is contrary to the objectives of the school vis a vis educating persons to be able to practice as members of the health care delivery team.[15]

Nevertheless, practitioners, teachers and students established their qualities by way of contrasts. That could promote a reaction. A fourth year student said: 'What really annoys me is when the lecturers are carrying on about physios as if we should be throwing spears at them'.

Most students participated in the condemnations. They spent a lot of time together in clinics, often with their supervisors present, talking, reading and writing up case notes between patient visits. Registered medical practitioners and physiotherapists came in for many passing shots, delivered wittily, sarcastically, or seriously, to an audience nodding in agreement or shaking heads in the formula of resigned but continuing amazement that such things still happened. On one occasion, stories were being exchanged about the bad things that doctors had done to patients and the important things they had left undone. After a while, the supervisor, who had added to the catalogue of horrors, brought the discussion to a halt: 'We've got to stop kicking our comrades in the medical profession!'.

The comrades influenced official actions. The order of the day was inter-professional concord based on the mutual recognition of valid healing works. Therefore confrères who stimulated external antagonism by way of their beliefs and actions had to be repudiated. Having stated their anti-denigration policy, teachers in the chiropractic sciences department went on to affirm that it was necessary 'to dissociate the school from questionable techniques, anti-medical and cultistic movements'. Not infrequently, however, students might interpret the school's stance as constraining teachers. One complained, 'They have all these successful things they do but the school won't let them tell us because they are supposed to be unscientific'. And another said, 'It's quite frustrating and negative here. The staff are not allowed to tell of the cures they make in practice. They are always cutting chiropractic down'.

Cultistic systems-mongers (as they were called by those who considered themselves to be scientific) were even more of a problem than the straights. Sacro-occipital technique (SOT) adherents were chief amongst them. 'Blocking' is typically associated with SOT practice. Rather than adjusting by the use of manual force, wedges are positioned under the recumbent body to achieve a gravitationally assisted pressure or torque.

Blocking might have as much to commend it as many another technique. It was safe. Nearly all physical therapists used the longitudinal application of force, or traction, for the treatment of certain musculo-skeletal conditions. What, then, made SOT less acceptable? Opponents criticised practitioners of it for: making inflated and unsubstantiated claims; maintaining a rigid diagnostic scheme; denying established chiropractic principles and procedures; being unprepared to conduct research and controlled trials; and being doctrinaire. It got back to what was scientific. The elaborate constructs of SOT theory — a sort of dialectical metabolism involving the cranium and the sacrum by way of the cerebro-spinal fluid — were considered 'way out' by critics in the school. The dean told me that SOT practitioners ought to be banned 'because [SOT] won't stand up in a court of law and because it is unscientific'. All sides, including the SOT practitioners, maintained that reason and science were on their side.

The practitioner organisation (SOTO) encouraged and subsidised student attendance at its certification seminars. The school preached sweat and tears as the conditions for passage through the course but announcements for introductory SOT sessions said that free pizza and beers would follow.[16] Students had other reasons for attending. SOT practitioners were stimulating. A fifth year who was about to undertake a SOT course told me: 'I must say the SOT people are so positive, so enthusiastic — it's the philosophy. A lot of students want that'. Another fifth year student said of SOT: 'They don't teach it here in the school because it's unscientific but, by gee, it works alright!'. Then there was employment. The SOTO told students:

S.O.T. chiropractors are among the most successful in Australia and overseas. Most of our experienced people are willing to share their time and experiences with you, if you are genuinely interested to learn, by providing Field Work places and Associateships so you are not left out on a limb once the umbilical cord of your college has been severed.[17]

The firm believers were trying to secure the continuity and growth of SOT by highlighting its advantages and by an active recruitment campaign. A number of teachers and students told me that the SOT plan was to 'stack' the student body with sponsored adherents. The SOT chairman had written: 'I have a plan. Let's fill every place at the two chiropractic colleges [i.e. Phillip and the Sydney college] with students who have come through S.O.T. practices'.[18] He went on to suggest that in the following year every SOT practitioner should have at least one patient accepted into chiropractic college and should plan on having one accepted every other year after that (as well as sponsoring students for the SOT-conducted seminars).

Nearly everybody thought that patients who had experienced the benefits of chiropractic made good students and suggesting a chiropractic career to them was entirely proper. But proselytising was construed as a takeover attempt when enemies did it. SOT was often talked about as an invasive danger and its practitioners were represented as chiropractic seducers. The dean abhorred the evangelising:

> They make a big effort to attract students. They actually have been seen handing money to students. They come up to them at conferences and make their acquaintance and show great interest in them . . . As a matter of fact, we have been thinking of changing the first year chiropractic principles course to introduce more stringent thinking, a more critical approach to the various theories.

A teacher (and early graduate of the school) said:

> The feverish excitement of SOT is influenced by the last person who brought you lunch! . . . They used to wine and dine the students, light their cigars with twenty dollar notes and blow their minds. When [the dean] came, he said it was all bullshit and didn't elaborate. But we came to see why. It was completely unscientific.

According to another graduate, SOT was the devil incarnate when he was a student: '[The dean] is very concerned to find a reason for what his enemies are doing and it's a standard one — it's the money, they are in it for the money — it's his standard way of opposing.

Important figures in the early history of the school were associated with SOT and it had been practised in the clinics. Once again, the 1981 transfer of education from the ICC to Phillip heralded a change in attitude. At the start of the following year, chiropractic sciences staff were still talking about attending SOT seminars wherever possible (the practitioner association allowed them to do so free of charge). The dean was to write asking for the honouring of an agreement that the association only teach the technique to students in fourth or fifth years:

> It was also felt that it may be advantageous if Clinical Board of Review decided that they would not authorise the practice of S.O.T. in the College Clinics until the student has met all of his patient quota requirement in the clinic, and has also passed Clinical Practicum IV.[19]

SOT was to be subsumed rather than excluded. Wedging procedures 'as used in sacro-occipital technique' were included in technique classes in 1983.[20] Later in the year, and on the dean's recommendation, the clinical board of review decided that SOT should be incorporated as an integral part of the undergraduate programme because:

a) a significant percentage of students and practitioners are actively involved with this system of practice. The Institute should therefore protect its own interests by accepting that its graduates would be competent to make decisions about the technique in terms of the integrated approach taught in the school.

b) it is only reasonable that students be afforded education in systems of practice in the undergraduate programme that provides them with a professional education.[21]

An important distinction was introduced. There were scientific techniques and there were others of proven benefit though their mode of action was poorly understood. The chiropractic sciences department decided that when the latter were taught in the undergraduate programme, 'it should be made quite clear to students that these are techniques proven on an empirical clinical basis without offering explanations for the mode of action'.[22]

SOT practitioners maintained that their approach was a chiropractic advance. 'In many cases', the association's newsletter said in an item directed to students, 'S.O.T. begins where ordinary manipulative techniques leave-off'.[23] After a school free-time introduction to SOT, a student told the presenter that it seemed SOT was going away from mainstream chiropractic, 'that is, adjusting with hands'. 'Yes' the practitioner replied:

that's true, it does move away from classical adjusting but not at a tangent from chiropractic — it *incorporates* chiropractic . . . The wholistic approach of SOT is chiropractic in that it relates to the nervous system and keeping it in balance.

SOT was not merely another technique but (in its purest expression) an alternative chiropractic. Practitioners of it had to be authorised in order to be acceptable. The association president told me:

SOTO does not teach SOT at either of the two Australian [chiropractic] colleges and will not do so without having control of the course material. We also do not sanction SOT being taught by anyone other than a fully certified SOT Instructor at the colleges or anywhere else . . . We do not sanction the use of SOT within the college clinics and would require a certified Instructor in attendance at all times for that to occur.[24]

While many straight and SOT concepts overlapped (and were equally repugnant to school leaders), it was not just ideas that had to be kept out but the SOT *system*. On the other side, protagonists of SOT believed the school repudiated them and at the same time adopted imperfect versions of their practices. In other words, the school was considered to have fallen into a merely empirical approach by detaching operations like blocking from their theoretical foundations. In just the same way, chiropractors and osteopaths believed registered medical practitioners and physiotherapists had stolen manipulative therapy without any proper education in or understanding of it; and traditional acupuncturists thought likewise about those doctors, physiotherapists and chiropractors who had taken up needling.

IF IT EVER CAME TO A COURT OF LAW

That chiropractic was a safe alternative to the excesses of drug therapy and radical surgery was held out as one of its principal claims to recognition. By the same token, the danger allegations of powerful critics had their influence on teaching. Great emphasis was placed on what could go wrong if techniques were inexpertly applied; and when something did go wrong, the readiness of enemies to publicise it was used to demonstrate a risk to the occupation. A teacher began one fourth year class with comments about medical alertness to chiropractic failings. Then he presented a summary of manipulative risks and contraindications. He said it was important to note that 'the reporting of these very rare accidents is used to malign chiropractic because they are given prominence in the papers, therefore we should be very careful'. A lengthy outline of the risks of established medical treatment followed (along the lines of the criticisms in Taylor's *Medicine Out of Control* (1979)). The teacher continued:

> They [the doctors] say that the risk of chiropractic is totally unacceptable. If there is one chiropractic accident it is across the front pages of every paper. But they don't know the dangers of prescribing practices of their simple therapies.

He said physiotherapists thought they had built up a body of evidence that the chiropractic thrust was the problem. There was no evidence that this was so 'but if you go to court, they can hold that against you. You should take every precaution to avoid risk because the risk is a major criticism of us'.

Thus, sound clinical behaviour was necessary to avoid putting the patient *and* the profession at risk. Also students were advised to protect themselves. If they used techniques like SOT then they could end up the legal creek without a paddle. One of the school's administrative staff explained to me:

> The school has certain rules, for example the one about only using school-taught techniques, because [the dean] says that if it came to a court of law he would have to be able to get up and say that the student was operating within the regular framework — that if the student was *not* then the case would be shaky.

Given all that students heard about oppositional representations of chiropractic as intrinsically dangerous, they were altogether aware of the need to be careful. As against this, the practitioner association told students how advantageous it was to have SOT in their bag of tricks. The techniques were popular with patients and 'It also keeps you out of the malpractice areas of chiropractic'.[25] Each side used the law argument against the other. But students could imagine that leaders emphasised safety because they feared ending up in court themselves. A fourth year student was commenting on the school's technique restrictions: 'When you hear [the dean] talking he is so cautious with everything. I suppose he has to be because he would have to face the courts or the media if anything went wrong'.

The possibility of court action bespoke other dangers. Males had to be careful in their treatment of female patients. The dean was giving a technique class: 'Watch where you put your hands! You don't want to get sued!'.

The readiness of enemies to seize examples of injury or death, as the NH&MRC had done with the coronial inquiry, led to the promotion of conservative treatment approaches. A teacher was discussing heart conditions with his fourth year acupuncture class. He was serious and ironic:

> I want to give it to you in TCM of course, but cardiac is a dicey area. You don't want any cardiac arrests on the table if you can avoid it. As in TCM, so in western medicine — everything can affect the heart, in the end. You have to approach it rather carefully. Hearts are rather dangerous and because TCM is powerful medicine you can stuff it up if you are not careful . . . Sort out the medical side first, ring the doctor first. Indeed *harass* the doctor. I refer to chapter 5 of the NH&MRC working party report — 'Acupuncture, Health and the Market Place' — a curious locution!

Students might end up acting so cautiously that they defeated the intention. Despite all that was said about established medical treatment risks and chiropractic safety, students could quickly send patients off to registered medical practitioners whenever they had the slightest doubt. The following exchange occurred when fifth years were using a case to practice for their final clinical oral exams:

Q. What would you do next?

A. I'd monitor him closely for any signs.

Q. How soon would you have him come back to see you?

A. I would have him go and see a G.P. next day!

Some even became reluctant to apply *standard* thrusting procedures and to steer clear of areas like the cervical spine. Without meaning to do so, the school gave them a stimulus to adopt 'safe' techniques like SOT in their subsequent practice. A student returned to the work room very upset after a patient had an adverse treatment reaction. She explained to the others present 'I ran my hand down the thoracic spine and said to her — 'did [another student who had previously treated the patient] adjust you here?' — and she said 'yes' so I adjusted and she freaked out! The student had come back to get an activator gun — a spring-loaded device that delivered a quick and very slight force through a rubber-tipped shaft. The gun was typically used by Activator practitioners, whose diagnostic and technique system was proscribed. However, the school had modified its stance by adopting the equipment: like SOT wedges, the gun had been detached from its system and allowed in clinics. The student returned after completing treatment and one of the supervisors (who had been observing) came in with a book interleaved with carbon paper:

> Supervisor: There's a possibility you've caused a fracture. We'd better write up a report.
>
> Student: You saw it, I thrusted very gently. I asked — 'has [the other student] adjusted you here before?' — you heard, she said 'yes'.
>
> Supervisor: What we've got to do is protect ourselves. [Another supervisor] gave you the O.K. to adjust. You gave a good adjustment.
>
> Student: Do you really think I caused her injury?
>
> Supervisor: When she got up off the table she was very tender. We've got to record it, just in case. It's better to be safe than sorry. We've got to be very careful.
>
> Student: You note that after that I used the activator?
>
> Supervisor: Yes, after.
>
> Student: Maybe she's a pretty tense person.
>
> Supervisor: She'll respond to a lot of massage, moddle-coddling, the activator. If she's tense she'll remain tense. It's better to have it written down than not reported at all.
>
> Student: It's taught me a lesson — never to presume what another clinician has done.
>
> Supervisor: It was a nice adjustment. Technique-wise, it was a nice adjustment.

When the supervisor departed after completing the report, the others joked about the incident but the student remained shaken. Later, she told me 'I really love a technique called SOT and I'll probably practice it when I get out of here. It's not forceful. It's a technique that's very useful for allergies, lower back pain and other things. I've had a lot of success with it'.

As a senior student reflected:

> Isn't it strange, you spend five years learning in the college but between a third and a half go out and within six months they are

involved with SOT. It seems that people go for it because it's an integrated step-by-step system, it hangs together . . . The school thinks it's doing these things [restricting SOT] for our protection but, really, they are keeping us from access to things we should have.

GETTING OUT

During their stay in clinics, students accommodated to conflicts about techniques and uncertainties about their careers. The testimony of practitioners — those people who were out there in the 'real' world — took on a new importance in defining sustaining occupational qualities. Nowhere was this the more evident than at a very well-attended school philosophy evening. One of the student organisers attended a Whole Health Institute seminar and she considered the speakers were so good that the students should hear them:

> [The dean] says we take a wholistic view in the course but it's not so. We spend so much time on science studies on the one hand and technique on the other there is no time for the sort of discussion of the whole person. The course is symptom oriented, musculo-skeletal oriented, so much so that the students have no opportunity to develop the whole-health approach.

The dean begged off attending. Revival meetings were not to his taste. A teacher introduced the four speakers. The first said he believed strongly 'in the connection between that power without and the intelligence within the body, within the cell. Homeostasis, that's another name for it'. Andrew Taylor Still likened the operations of bodies to cities. This chiropractor used a similar metaphor:

> When you look at their function, the cells are very much working in order, the family of cells. I think the Innate Intelligence gives us that order. Look at the heart: can you go out to the hardware store and buy a pump that is likely to work for 70, 80, 90 years? It's the same intelligence that works to keep the body in order. The liver is a marvellous chemical factory. The kidneys are a sewerage system. The body does these things automatically. How automatically? Again, it is Innate Intelligence. All of this put together makes a wonderful body . . . When you go out to practise it is necessary to realise there is something more to life than earning money. My experience is that if you do the right thing about the patient, the

love, concern and empathy, my experience is that you'll not have any problems about the money . . . Always remember that shining star of chiropractic — that's what you always must keep your eye on.

If they had been there to hear, how contemptuous the secularists would be of such evocations of the numinous! But the large student audience was transfixed. The next speaker, a Phillip graduate, was the star of the evening. She touched the chord of student experience:

When I got to PIT in 1982, we got philosophy. We got tone and vitalism. The next lecture was the 32 principles. I thought: what *bullshit*! I thought: I know what chiropractic is doing is right and what chiropractic is doing is helpful; I know the body has an intelligence that is far greater than the sum of its parts. I knew this intuitively. In fifth year I felt a wreck. You go to school to help people and they turn you into a screaming heap!

A student asked about her practice:

It's really exciting. I hope to make a healing centre out of what is a multi-disciplinary clinic. I have been dabbling in homeopathy. I have a crystal, I also have a crystal in my office. I use whatever seems right for the person, be it rationally sound or off with the fairies! If it works, if it seems to work for *me* then I'll do it! . . . Most people don't want to know about your beliefs until the pain has gone away! Healing takes time. What you have to do is provide the right healing atmosphere.

Another asked her whether the healing atmosphere was the placebo effect or her effect on the patient. She parried: 'The placebo effect on the patient or on me?' It was a significant point. In one way or another, exemplary practitioners told students *they* had to feel good about chiropractic, have the flow, be healed themselves if they were to be effective healers.

The message here was as inspiring as Reggie Gold's, yet different. The healing possibilities were endless. Straight chiropractic was amongst them but far from the only one. None of the speakers argued from a technique or system position. B.J. was not mentioned, though another speaker, also a Phillip graduate, affirmed that the philosophy of chiropractic used deductive reasoning ('It's O.K. to use inductive reasoning as a cross-reference'). As he said, getting the body to function better was something the body itself did: 'My job as a chiropractor is to allow the brain to get in contact with the rest of the body, and that's it'.

These were heady messages and they cut across the official position. It was not that the students fell prey to madcaps, as leaders supposed. Rather, the school's own strictness about scientific regularity, ambiguity about the use of varieties of technique, and the imminence of a liberating departure from the school made the therapeutic possibilities imaginable. The response of many is captured in a student newsletter item following another forum (held outside the school) where practitioners of various alignments testified about chiropractic:

> It was great as a student to see that chiropractic is more than just applications of anatomy and physiology or about making money. It was wonderful to see the enthusiasm of the speakers for chiropractic and how strongly they believed in it. Such enthusiasm was infectious.
>
> As students, the Forum gave us a positive boost and made us realise that there is light at the end of the tunnel!![26]

Prior to fourth year, students did not stand before patients and decide what to do. Now that had happened and each of them, armed with a certainty about chiropractic, had to make an uncertain choice about the treatment to give. Early in her fourth year a student told me (with the others present agreeing):

> They [the teachers] present us with a lot of techniques — you know, 'if this doesn't work, try this and if that doesn't work, try this' . . . There's a lot of people in the course who will become straight chiros — that's what they want to be!

Another, a third year student, made a connection between the antagonism to chiropractic, the importance of a scientific foundation and the lack of a definitive school approach:

> I came through the feeder course [an interstate arrangement where students undertook a science degree with anatomy and physiology majors alongside some profession-arranged chiropractic education]. [A chiropractic teacher in the feeder course] put us very firmly in the line of scientific musculo-skeletal medicine. But there are so many quacks in this profession! And we are being squeezed out. Will there be a chiropractic occupation in future? Here at PIT they

seem to teach everything — there is no clear basis for us, it's not at all clear what happens to us — we are threatened on all sides.

What emerged was a student distinction between the school expectation and the professional condition. One fifth year student concluded: 'In order to be a chiropractor you have to be an opinionated, cantankerous person who gets out of college and develops your own technique'.

The view that science, clarity about the technical applications and enthusiasm for chiropractic were not sufficiently combined by the school, already strong by third year, consolidated in the clinical years. Students agreed that they should be scientific, of course, but many also believed that science was not enough, by itself, to carry the practice of healing. Where was the guide? The students knew many things but now they had to act.

They contrasted their experience in studying science with the healing philosophy that was supposed to distinguish their occupation. A fifth year student said:

> What is most troublesome is the way basic sciences dominate the course. It means that the study of chiropractic is put last, it's the thing you do a few days before the exams. You'd probably know more about chiropractic history and theory from your studies than I do. It's a bit of a disappointment, really, but I suppose that's the way it has to be.

The official school hitched its star to science because science was the right way and because alliance with it made for reputability in much the same was as dress made for professionalism. Thus the dean told the executive, in discussing a possible alteration to the naming of degrees in chiropractic and osteopathy after the introduction of a degree in human biology as the first part of a double degree programme:

> I'd favour 'Science' at the end — 'Bachelor of Chiropractic Science' and 'Bachelor of Osteopathic Science', like 'Bachelor of Dental Science' and 'Bachelor of Veterinary Science' — because people think we are quacks.

But many students thought healing involved something in addition. A fifth year said that when he took up study again in his early thirties he had been very enthused about science and thought it explained all. Now he believed there had to be 'something over, on top of science, Innate Iintelligence, call it what you will . . . whatever you call it, Innate Intelligence or Qi, it's much the same — it's the "grey box" of explanation'.

As another chiropractic teacher suggested to his class:

Generally it's supposed [in science] that if you put forward an idea the onus is on the proponent to establish why. But you could put it the other way around: is there any reason why not? Chiropractic was proposing ideas in a field that had no body of knowledge itself. At the time of Palmer there was no musculo-skeletal body of knowledge so it faced a lot of resistance because people were unfamiliar with the concepts.

As they approached the end of the course it was rare to find a student without a catalogue of resentments about the school. One told me: 'I'll spend the next month trying to purge myself of these feelings rather than be like my friend who, a year later [i.e. after passing fifth year], still can't even physically bear to drive up to the place'.

I asked senior students and graduates what they had to do in order to get through the course. Nearly all chiropractic students responded with versions of the 'satisfy the teachers' theme:

You relate what you do to what you think they want. If you are doing something for [a teacher] then it has to be exactly right, 'yes' or 'no'. But if it's [another teacher] then the thing can be much woollier because for him there's no right answer.

Submission was necessary. A fourth year student answered my enquiry by saying 'Co-operate. A senior student told me when I was in first year: "co-operate to graduate". What you've got to do is take all the stuff they throw at you.'

Teachers themselves, those who had passed through the school, shared the opinion:

Conform. The school is held together with an administrative system that doesn't make sense, so what you've got to do is conform. The rules are used on a 'needs' basis, so that when something is not liked or wrong you look up the rules and find one and invoke it.

Compliance was far from entire and it generated a reaction. Another school graduate (and clinic supervisor) said:

My body learned to adjust to the school, to take everything that came. What you have to do is lie down flat and not kick. I kicked in the earlier years . . . The staff put pressure on you and you put pressure back. You have to find ways of getting around things. If we weren't together as a group, I don't know what we would have done . . . I remember when we had all these urine analyses outstanding so what we did was get together and make them all up. In the end, you get so that nothing disturbs you. Another exam — you just do it and get out as quickly as you can. You learn not to make difficulties.

Osteopathy students, then in their fourth year, responded similarly. 'Suffer', one said, 'You have to wreck yourself to do this course'. Others agreed with her. They were a much smaller group — there were eleven of them — and their solidarity was important: 'It's the unity of the group. We've developed a strong unity about helping each other out, copying notes if you can't be there and so on'.

The earlier three years became remote, academic. The world of the clinic was much more like being in the 'real' world but it was at just this time that students became most vocal about 'getting into the real world'. They meant escaping the bondage to the school. One told me (immediately following the fifth year finals) 'I just decided to pass. I had to pass to get rid of this big white elephant I'm tied to so I can get on with my life'. Another fifth year student said:

It's sad to be ending this way. It could be better. They are so inconsistent with the rules. They can hide behind them or insist on them as they wish. It's repressive: you can follow the rules and it doesn't lead to any recognition but others don't follow them and that's ignored.

At one of the 'departure' dinners, a third explained: 'To tell you the truth, I'm so pleased to be getting out of the place. I suppose I should feel elated at getting to the end of the course but I don't. I just want to be away as soon as I can'.

I asked many chiropractic and osteopathy students whether they would come back to undertake postgraduate research courses in the school. None wanted to do so and only a very few saw research (however desirable it was for the occupation) as a career for them. One said:

It's been a long time. It'll be seven years by the time I finish [the student had begun by taking a science degree with an anatomy major]. My car is stuffed, my clothes are getting tatty and the debts are mounting up. There's no way that I would want to do research straight away.

The more usual reason for rejecting the possibility was the desire to escape school control. With heavy irony, another said: 'Chiropractors deserve to go out and earn a lot because they have been through hell for five years!'. There was a mocking stock response students gave when they aired their complaints about the school to each other: 'So what do you want for free?'. Graduation, when it came, was a ceremony of formal release. Yet education marked them: whatever turns their practice might take, the school remained, for all its imperatives, as their distinctive badge within the profession.

Notes

(Unless otherwise noted, documents are from the School of Chiropractic and Osteopathy archives and working files).

1. Kelly, B. 'From the President's Pen', *The Axis* 2, 30 April 1990.
2. 'SWOT Analysis and Strategy Plan in Relation to Amalgamation with La Trobe University', discussed at school executive committee, 31 July 1989.
3. 'Admissions Selection Policies and Procedures for 1989 Intake', 5 October 1988, p. 3.
4. 'Objectives and Implementation Guidelines for the Admissions Interview Panels', n.d. (October 1988), p. 3.
5. 'Panel Interview Form' and 'Convenor Interview Form', 19 August 1987.
6. Objectives and Implementation Guidelines ... [Ref. 4], p. 7.
7. Compiled from acupuncture college records. Those who did not indicate current employment are included in the remainder percentage. Excluded from the age calculation are a few applicants who did not give birth dates.
8. 'Equity', n.d., attached to memo from Gray, R. (assistant director, planning and educational services), 6 October 1989.
9. Institute Resources Committee, Phillip Institute of Technology, 'Participation of Women in Institute Courses', n.d. (September 1989).
10. In 1989, 38% of the successful chiropractic applicants and 59% of the successful osteopathy applicants were female. Rates varied over the years:

	1982	1983	1984	1985	1986	1987	1988	1989
Chiropractic (%)	28	23	34	25	37	29	32	38
Osteopathy (%)	-	-	-	-	33	52	28	59

'Percentage of Successful Applicants: Gender Distribution', School of Chiropractic and Osteopathy, 5 May 1989.
11. Extracted from school statistics.
12. Excell, L. (Vice-President of the student union) to Kelly, B. (President of the CSA), 16 May 1990. Reproduced in *The Axis* 4, June 1990.
13. 'From the President's Pen', *The Axis* 4, June 1990.

14. There were 102 women and 204 men enrolled in the chiropractic course in 1989. Details by year were:

Year	Chiropractic		Osteopathy	
	Male	Female	Male	Female
1	48	29	11	15
2	46	24	16	8
3	40	18	8	6
4	35	21	6	5
5	35	10	-	-
Totals	204	102	41	34

Extracted from Table 2 in 'Annual Report to the Commission on Accreditation of the Australasian Council on Chiropractic and Osteopathic Education', School of Chiropractic and Osteopathy, March 1990.

15. Minutes, Chiropractic Sciences department, 1984.

16. 'Free Introductory Offer to S.O.T.' Announcement for 21 February 1990 lecture in common free time and 24 February 'hands-on' demonstration of SOT at a private clinic.

17. *Chairman's Corner*, Newsletter of the Sacro-Occipital Technique Organisation, December 1987, p. 2.

18. *Chairman's Corner* . . . , April 1988, p. 1.

19. Minutes, Chiropractic Sciences meeting, 17 March 1982.

20. Minutes, Chiropractic Sciences meeting, 9 February 1983.

21. Reported in Minutes, Chiropractic Sciences meeting, 29 June 1983.

22. Minutes, Chiropractic Sciences meeting, 15 June 1983.

23. *Chairman's Corner* . . . , December 1987, p. 2.

24. Letter from Leyonhjelm, K. to the author, 12 June 1989.

25. *Chairman's Corner* . . . , December 1987, p. 2.

26. Karagiannis, J. and Tornatora, B., *The Axis* 2, April 1990.

X

CASTE, CLASS AND THE HEALING OCCUPATIONS

Relinquishment of caste is the outward and visible sign of the realisation than one's true state is 'unclassified', that one's role or person is simply conventional, and that one's true nature is 'no-thing' and 'no-body'.

(Alan Watts, *The Way of Zen*, 1972, 64.)

INTRODUCTION

Chiropractors, osteopaths and traditional acupuncturists had far from given up espousing medical revivals, though in their teaching institutions the emphasis had shifted to scientific reputability and partnership in the offer of medical care.

A wider question is discussed in this final chapter. The persistent denial and denigration of the three medicines has been described but how is it to be explained? Two theories are discussed. According to the first, healing occupations are arranged in a caste-like system. On the second, the class structure of modern capitalist society is replicated in the disposition of medical occupations.

I am concerned to avoid embedding chiropractors, osteopaths and traditional acupuncturists in an analytic scheme that yields their actions and convictions as the effects of determining social formations and processes. Rather than classifying them, I have attempted to show the ways in which they live out their own formulations of occupational place and purpose. I do attempt to move beyond the immediate preoccupations of students and teachers in order to comprehend fixities of place and restrictions on social relations between medicines. Chiropractors, osteopaths and traditional acupuncturists not only located themselves (and framed their internal differences) by reference to distinctive beliefs and practices but were, in turn, so categorised, especially by physiotherapists and registered medical practitioners. Their generalisations were not of a piece, fully espoused, or steadily held.

One could easily find physiotherapists and doctors who were quite supportive of chiropractors and the rest, or who altered their opinions on closer acquaintance. Nevertheless, occupational associations relayed the same characterisations over decades. The AMA had much the same thing to say about chiropractic in 1975-77 (at the time of the Victorian and federal inquiries), in 1985-86 to the Medicare review committee and the Victorian parliamentary social development committee, and in its 1992 position paper. Nor was there much to distinguish between the interpretations of orthodox medical purposes and actions in chiropractic association responses.

For all the advances they made in gaining higher education and government regulation, the overall situation of the three occupations — that is, their social positioning in relation to other medical groups, to registered medicine in particular — had but little changed. The proof was in the upholding of barriers to collaboration (as indicated by the lack of referrals for treatment from doctors), to hospital engagement, and to full participation in public health insurance arrangements. Chiropractors, osteopaths and traditional acupuncturists were still shut out of the game. One might put this down to prejudice or to the self-interest that ideology masks but the consistent enforcement of isolation demands some wider and less personalised understanding.

I start with a discussion of the systematic distinctions represented by caste and class. I then submit that the identity and relation of healing occupations, their meanings for those engaged in them, are established in the figurative intermingling of notions about bodily and medical organisation and functioning. The subject matter of medicine and the social objects of medical groups coalesce to express these meanings and to confirm their rightness.

CASTE AND CLASS

Caste and class theorists are sometimes inclined to forget that they are attempting to convey one or other of many possible understandings of social life, not representing it as it is. In other words, they overlook the fact that their terminological constructions are devised and employed to conceive a field; instead, they purport to demonstrate its essential or intrinsic characteristics. 'Caste' and 'class' are used here suggestively. The former is intended to draw attention to the believed or organic order — that in use by the participants — and the latter brings out the mechanics of organisation in the received social order.

A caste interpretation is attractive because it captures the influence of affective as well as structural elements in the relations of health occupations — not only the legal sanctions but also what De Vos (1967, 78) called the visceral sanctions that keep people apart in a caste system. Caste draws attention to the presupposition of an entrenched hierarchical arrangement, to the fixity of places in it, and to the values and attitudes that sustain it. There is a sense of inevitability about caste relations, whether historically determined or understood by subscribers as expressing the fitness of a social order:

> Castes and guilds arise from the action of the same natural law, that regulates the differentiation of plants and animals into species and varieties, except that, when a certain degree of development has been reached, the heredity of castes and the exclusiveness of guilds are ordained as laws of society (Marx, 1954 vol.1, 321).

The caste system is contained, tautological and inescapable. It specifies the allowable range and form of convivial relations through the symbolic oppositions of the sacred and the profane, the safe and the unsafe, what is pure and what is defiling. The organising principle of caste, religious in the Indian case and scientific in the health order, is expressed by proscriptions and rituals governing conduct.

Work is ranked by its cleanness, a notion with powerful health associations. A degree of concurrent ritual immunity is assumed by higher order castes and healers in their potentially defiling or infective contacts (for an example of the inverse relationship between medical rank and the use of caps, gowns and masks for protection against TB 'contagion', see Roth, 1957). As Mary Douglas argued, the idea of dirt as matter out of place implies two conditions: a set of ordered relations and a contravention of that order. Dirt, then, is not an isolated event: 'Whenever there is dirt there is system . . . In short, our pollution behaviour is the reaction which condemns any object or idea likely to confuse or contradict cherished classifications' (Douglas, 1979, 35-36). Caste, then, is 'a symbolic system, based on the image of the body, whose primary concern is the ordering of a social hierarchy' (Douglas, 1979, 125).

In extending the idea of purity to the professions, Abbott (1981, 823-824) drew on caste as a cultural system. Rather than being based on income, power, client status, or task complexity (all of which failed to accord consistently with intra-professional rankings), status was a function of professional purity. The refinement and removal of direct human complexity and difficulty left problems that were professionally defined or definable. As in caste, 'The clear is more pure than the amorphous, the definite more pure than the ambiguous'. Features of work which were disparaged and led to low status — association with the occupationally confounding messiness of human affairs — were, paradoxically, the foundations of public esteem which came from effective contact with disorder. Therefore, drawing back into purity was a professional regression which opened the way for new professions and old rivals to take over the dirty work and capture the public charisma associated with it.

As we have seen, alternative practitioners affirm their repute by saying that they deal successfully with people who have turned to them as a last resort. This connection with frequent but little understood, poorly defined and intractable conditions establishes an outcaste ranking for the alternatives even as it secures their clientele. Statements about the liabilities of contact with alternative practitioners, the prospect of being injured or even killed by them, are not simply devices intended to turn patients away from the alternatives. The conviction of danger evidences the systemic power of a fixed medical order; and what is impure, according to that order, is defiling.

An earlier example, the NH&MRC acupuncture reports (Westerman, 1988; 1989), indicates the potency of a caste interpretation. Science was invoked to exorcise unnacceptable practitioners. The infective potential of contact with them was contrasted with the hygienic practices of registered medicine. 'Lay' and 'non-medical' descriptors underlined the exclusion. Through their unscientific, unsafe characterisation, working party members enacted their understanding of the fitting order by denying the traditional acupuncturists.

Any cross-cultural utilisation of caste faces the difficulty that rules of endogamy and of birth ascription are absolute in the Indian system of caste relations (in its idealised version though not, of course, in its contemporary operation, for the members of outcaste groups can refuse to accept their 'ordained' place). The situation of Negroes in the southern United States appeared to conform to this requirement and caste was the central interpretative figure in a number of earlier studies of American race relations, such as Dollard's *Caste and Class in a Southern Town* (1937, reprinted in 1957).

While caste and class were 'ways of dividing people according to the behaviour expected of them in society' (1957, 61-62), Dollard used caste exclusively to indicate the organisation of and justification for the line between the races. Caste seemed 'to be modelled on the patriarchal family with its possessive prerogatives of the male'. It was a categoric and emotionally charged distinction necessarily involving binary hierarchies: classes existed within the societies on either side of the caste divide (p. 83). Both caste and class were systems of social stratification but caste, as W. Lloyd Warner had proposed (1936, 234), could be further defined by the limits on movement between groups and by the prohibitions on inter-group marriage.

Dollard showed the instrumentality of caste in safeguarding and perpetuating a moral and status order. Others who have used caste cross-culturally have followed this approach. For example, Berreman (1960, 123; 1967, 49) considered the essential similarity between caste and race systems to be the maintenance of institutionalised inequality based on convictions of differences in intrinsic worth.

Our understanding of health occupations also can be informed by thinking about them in terms of a system of caste relations. Anderson (1981, 158) maintained that even though the ordering of health work failed to meet a strict caste definition, the opportunities for inter-group movement, though available in principle, were strikingly less common in the medical world than in the occupational structure as a whole. Health employment also exhibited many other features of a caste-like system, especially in the rating by orthodox practitioners (that is, the members of 'higher castes') of chiropractors as untouchables. 'A hard-working person cannot leave his caste to join one higher in the system' but whole groups might aspire to a changed status by using a high caste as a model: 'To do so, the members of a caste must convince everyone that they occupy a low position by mistake. They must argue that history somehow wrongly placed them in their ignominious position' (1981, 159). Chiropractors had imitated medical behaviour and appearance and had adopted the orthodox medical system of education. Nevertheless, the barriers of hostility remained and interaction was denied them. Anderson concluded that:

in striving for upward mobility [chiropractors] are impelled to imitate higher status doctors, yet are caught in a dilemma of cultural differentiation and caste regulation that closes off access to aspects of medical education that could facilitate their striving. Medical doctors, for their part, resist the growth of manual medicine within their own ranks. This they do, it would appear, more because manipulation functions as a symbol of despised caste status than because it fails to meet the needs of clinical practice (Anderson, 1981, 164).

In passing, upper caste imitation — Sanskritisation as it is called — bears comparison with what is generally termed professionalisation and is found in the upward striving conducted on behalf of all 'subsidiary' health occupations by their associations. Orthodox medicine provides the model for alternative health occupations too, but their outcaste status, with all that is implied about opposition to their securing recognition on even the lowest rungs of the caste ladder, is a formidable hurdle.

Despite the resistance, successful medical emulations do occur, as in the conversion of Californian osteopaths into registered medical practitioners. The shift was total: members were transformed as a group and on condition that they threw off all osteopathic identifications. Similarly, U. S. homeopaths were absorbed into a high status category. The decline of this medicine did not result from the conclusive discrediting of its theory. In 1903 the American Medical Association changed its rules in such a way that local medical societies were enabled to accept homeopaths. The fact that they had graduated from irregular colleges no longer precluded them: what was required was a recantation of adherence to an exclusive system of medicine (Kaufman, 1971, 155).

These instances demonstrate features of the health order. While individuals in one occupation may change their status by undertaking education for another, the position of an occupation as a whole is only altered by its merger with a more prestigious one. In which case, characteristics which formerly distinguished members — such as convictions of mission, singular practices, titles of rank and the occupational name — are removed and replaced by those of the superior group. Even in the Indian caste system, a changed status is not ruled out but the system remains and the possibilities of advancement are limited to submergence in an existing classification. This rigidity has led to attacks on the caste interpretation of health work.

In her thesis on the natural therapies in Australia, Wiesner (1983, 218) maintained that those who used caste or structural marginality theories condemned practitioners 'to an inflexible role as therapists and an unchangeable status. Community perceptions of the natural therapies and the involvement of their practitioners in the practice of holistic medicine refute such models'. She argued that a broad definition of caste minimised the significance of culturally specific features and additional terms had to be introduced to clarify the relationship between caste, as broadly conceived, and the class phenomenon. Anderson and Warner had failed to distinguish between the features of a social system, such as endogamy, and the social system itself with the practices actually followed in it (pp. 207-209). The Indian restriction on caste and outcaste group associations might not apply elsewhere, and:

> Equally troublesome in the case of chiropractors is the inference that their exclusion is grounded in notions of ritual impurity rather than the facts of occupational mobility. It is equally noteworthy, in passing, that Indian caste groups are occupationally complementary, not competitors.

Wiesner allowed there was some value in the use of the concepts of caste and untouchability but they only provided a relatively simple explanation of the failure of chiropractic to move beyond its label of fringe or alternative medicine. Instead, and based on the work of Klegon (1978), she identified the occurrence of a professionalising process with internal and external dynamics. The burden of her case was that while orthodox medical opposition continued to be formidable, the natural therapies had achieved an enhanced position through professionalising activity. Their entry as 'cohesive and ambitious professional groups' into the active arena of medical politics added impetus for change (p. 239).

This professionalisation model did not explain the failure of homeopathy and naturopathy to advance at all, the holding of chiropractic and osteopathy at the registration and higher education stage of their pursuits, and, most of all, the continued established medical repudiation of association with any of the alternatives, whatever their official gains. Her model amounted to a schematisation of the strategies used by occupational associations in endeavours to improve their own houses and to represent their causes to 'Wider Social Forces'.

Freidson (1988b, 76-77) suggested the transfer of training to higher education institutions and licensing were useful conditions for the development of an autonomous occupation, but 'that they are necessary conditions is moot; that they are sufficient conditions is plainly false'. In this respect, members of alternative and allied medical occupations are in the same boat: they secure professional attributes without necessarily advancing in rank. The signs of high caste are mistaken for the existence of it. In looking for recognition as full professions, nurses, occupational therapists, physiotherapists, and the rest, seek to escape their subordination. In comparison, even as the chiropractic, osteopathic and traditional acupuncture occupations have been changed by the pursuit of official recognition, the practitioners have held onto the autonomy that exclusion allowed them. Above everything else, their unpreparedness to cede primary patient contact rights has secured their independence.

Not only have the alternatives failed to realise the gains that are supposed to result from the adoption of professional marks but also the pursuit has heightened internal animosities. This is especially so when overly scientific preoccupations are considered to diminish the qualities that made the medicine into another and better answer in the first place. In denouncing counter-movements for selling out on their principles, a sociologist (Rose, 1979, 279) echoed a familiar criticism made by segments of chiropractic, osteopathy and traditional acupuncture:

> By observing the Sanskrit of science, a group of untouchables wishes to translate itself into a position within the caste system of science. Like Black Capitalists or Bourgeois Feminists, they do not wish to change the world — merely to join it.

I do not wish to question here whether professionalisation is a useful tool for analysis but whether it works. An occupation may secure its continuance by becoming registered and gaining a qualifying course of university instruction. Certainly, these achievements buttress the self-esteem of members and are advanced by them to evidence that they are the equals of the likes of doctors, as in the chiropractors' response (CAA, 1993) to their denunciation by the AMA.

Yet control structures and workplace relations are largely unaltered, key tasks are closely guarded, differentials in salaries and other employment advantages continue, and partnership status, the health care team idea, is more talked about by aspirants to it than realised in the operation of health care institutions. For all the intensity of professionalising endeavour, the relative occupational condition remains much the same.

In terms of professionalisation, interpretations of occupational movement, what caste brings out is the systematic articulation of individual and collective meanings. A status is tied to the group and the group is settled in a place. The individual strives for enhanced position through group pursuits. When the members of repudiated occupations take on attributes and customary behaviour associated with those in groups above them, they confuse, as Berreman put it (1967, 49), the idiom in which caste rank is expressed for the criteria by which it is conferred. The failure of professionalising activity to deliver the intended result can be understood in such terms: those in 'higher' groups justify their continued resistance by maintaining that certain essential features are still lacking. Alternative medicines always will be found lacking because the orthodox medical conviction is that nothing less than a regular medical education will do to qualify the practitioners of medicine. The diminishment of alternative occupations can be supplemented by drawing attention to the working-class antecedents of members, usually without the aid of evidence, but this is by way of reinforcing the characterisation rather than being central to it.

Willis (1983, 4) understood the division of labour in health care 'as a process based upon conflict; a struggle between occupations and between the sexes, not so much over occupational roles but over occupational territory or task domains'. He said that established medicine obtained its dominance as a pay-off for reproducing capitalist productive relations and maintaining the associated ideological hegemony. Therefore the politico-legal legitimation of a 'new' medicine involved a double system of patronage: having obtained its dominant position by exercising a state-conferred agency function, established medicine was enabled to sponsor or deny other medical occupations. The price of legitimation was acceptance of a subordinated or limited position (p.197; see also Miles-Tapping, 1985, who explained the Canadian relationship between established medicine and physiotherapy in similar terms).

In this tight, enclosed and dominative system how, then, can one explain the success of chiropractic and osteopathy in securing politico-legal legitimation despite the lack of scientific acceptance and established medical opposition? Given the capitalist agency function of medicine, this is a crucial question as Willis's argument seems to run counter to the result.

Willis said that to some extent the legitimacy of the state itself was at stake: 'the fact that so many people attended chiropractors meant that it could not be ignored and expected to go away' (p. 197). But more important was the growing compatibility of chiropractic knowledge with dominant class interests. If anything, chiropractic espoused more of an engineering approach to health than did established medicine: 'individuals are like machines which can be tinkered with to get back into good running order. And good running order means producing surplus value' (p. 198). Statutory recognition brought on, as it were, a chiropractic mimesis of established medicine. Willis said that the condition for its legitimation was that chiropractors abandoned their claim to be a complete alternative and instead were recognised as specialists in spinal manipulative therapy. They were limited, rather than subordinated, because they had retained their status as primary contact practitioners.

According to Willis, chiropractors had 'joined the ranks of the "organic intellectuals" of capitalist societies, becoming important agents of social control on behalf of capital in their own right' (p. 200). This metamorphosis was an artefact of his categories, themselves an expression of his theoretical scheme. If chiropractors succeeded in gaining registration and a state-accredited course, then, inevitably, they entered another class position and took on the functions definitionally associated with it. Chiropractors must have left one rank in order to join another. Yet never had there been an incongruity between chiropractic and the capitalist productive mode. Practitioners no more shifted from opposing to endorsing it than did osteopaths and traditional acupuncturists. Further, the new rank did not lead to altered relationships with other organic intellectuals: they continued to be isolated by them.

Established medicine surely relies on official support for its continued ascendancy. It hardly could be otherwise when the state is largely responsible for the funding, organisation and supervision of medical services. However, the capitalist productive mode becomes the unseen regulator when it is given explanatory primacy. And by extension of Willis's point about established medicine being a beneficiary of the capitalist system because of support for its maintenance, even the more recent State tolerance of alternative medicines can be explained: the gatekeeper function and the associated need for surveillance and control of the labour force are less important in times of high unemployment.

Ideology is an opaque surface that has to be stripped away in order to reveal the dominative mechanism. Willis was explicit about exposing the causal forces. He made an epistemological distinction between appearance and reality and spoke of using a theoretical scaffolding to order and analyse historical evidence:

The historical investigation then is concerned with the level of appearances . . . These appearances however derive from and are the effects of underlying structures, contradictory, fragmented and subject to transformation by struggle (such as class and gender) but essential nonetheless for the explanation of appearances (p. 214).

Appearances did not just obscure reality — they were an intentional smoke-screen: 'the state must protect the economic interests of the dominant class without appearing to do so' (p. 28); and: 'Medical dominance then rests upon state patronage, achieved through medicine's role in reproducing the relations of production and seeking to maintain bourgeois ideological hegemony' (p. 204). Everything verified this teleological interpretation, a failing Popper (1972, 34-37) detected in Marxist and psychoanalytic constructions. The theoretical scaffolding *was* the structure and created its own reality.

As Parkin observed (1979, 113), from a Marxist point of view, any given set of occupational strategies could 'in principle be understood as mere responses to the material pressures and forces set in play by the capitalist mode of production'. The difficulty with a pure class analysis, he also suggested (1974, 2), was that where class was defined by reference to dual, logically exhaustive categories it followed that antagonisms *within* any given category could not properly be understood as manifestations of conflict in the accredited sense. The vocabulary of class did not 'readily lend itself to the analysis of stratification and cleavage associated with membership in racial, ethnic, religious, and linguistic communities'. The healing occupations can be added to Parkin's list.

This stricture might not apply to all class explanations but only to those that rely on binary oppositions, as was the case with Willis. Other interpretations, such as the one advanced by Schumpeter (1955) and utilised by Ben-David (1963-1964), generate plausible accounts of a mobility that is achieved through the exploitation of new or previously overlooked activities. According to the former, 'For the duration of its collective life, or the time during which its identity may be assumed, each class resembles a hotel or an omnibus, always full, but always of different people' (Schumpeter, 1955, 126). The content of any 'upper class' was not merely modified but formed by the rise and decline of families, the more so in a capitalist industrial system, and was a matter 'of first creating a position which is then recognised to be a fact' (p. 132). The barriers to movement from one class to another were not different in kind, only in strength, to those impeding elevation within a class. But a new element was introduced, entirely absent in situations of intra-class movement (where a person might advance by being more successful than others in effecting cures, for example). It was 'to *do something altogether different* from what is, as it were, ordained to the individual' (p. 132).

Schumpeter's theory also can be applied to comprehend the appearance and growth of occupations that have not depended on the sponsorship of established medicine. Licensing and formal higher education corroborate their successful exploitation of previously ignored or neglected activities, like manipulation. This bears on the idea that legitimation follows on clinical success but does not assist in an understanding of the persistence of dismissiveness and exclusionary actions — 'the necessary idiom of conflict' in social relations that Parkin (1974, 13) associated with class explanations and that are not captured either in a caste interpretation. It will not do to use caste or class solely, by stretching definitions, or to establish class differentiations within the established and alternative medical spheres, and then resort to caste for an explanation of the chasm between them.

Dumont noted (1972, 287ff) that in its earlier American sociological use, caste was frequently taken to be an extreme case of class. He opposed the application of caste to American race relations because particular features were extracted from the whole Indian social system without establishing whether those that were chosen were sufficient to define it.

Since distinctions of honour and fitting social intercourse are what counts in medical relations, Weber's status group type (1978, 305-307), with its emphasis on successful occupational claims to esteem and monopolistic appropriation, is more apt. For Weber, caste was an example of status grouping in which 'the obligations and barriers . . . are intensified to the utmost degree' (1948: 405). Thus, 'As a 'status group', "caste" enhances and transfers this social closure into the sphere of religion, or rather of magic' (p. 408).

Dumont (1972, 290-291) was also critical of this approach, suggesting that Weber 'wanted to link up widespread ideas on the racial origin of the caste system with the exceptional situation of certain minority communities like Jews and Gypsies in Western societies'. Dumont's argument (1972, 71) was that the analysis of caste should begin with the overall theory of it and that caste could not be extracted from Indian culture (see also Dumont 1967, where he opposed reducing the 'ideal type of pure hierarchy' as found in India to a classified form of social stratification).

Once again, it is a matter of definition. Passin (1967, 329) concluded a symposium on comparative approaches to caste and race by saying that:

'Caste' can be defined in such a way that it does not occur even in India, or so that all the characteristics of the definition come together in only one single village somewhere in Andhra. It can also be defined in such a way that it occurs anywhere in the world. To some extent it is a matter of choice: for certain purposes it may be useful to limit the definition; for other purposes it may be useful to inspect the entire universe from the standpoint of certain criteria and see what we find.

In part, a difficulty arises when an ideal-type of caste is placed at one extreme on a continuum along which systems of social stratification are ranged (e.g. by Berreman, 1960, 121). The result is that caste and class become artificially separated on an oppositionally constructed dimension. Thus Berreman asserted (1967, 49, his italics) *'In a caste system an individual displays the attributes of his caste because he is a member of it. In a class system, an individual is a member of his class because he displays its attributes'*. The distinction is by no means so neat. Class is a lived classification as well as a means of socially locating groups of individuals by their possession of designated attributes. Likewise, caste, the exemplary case of an embracing scheme, has its principles theorised by commentators. The problem here is that analytic and supposedly objective devices also have meaning for those who are to be accounted by them.

Chiropractors, osteopaths and traditional acupuncturists have the general class attributes of established medical practitioners and physiotherapists and their relationship to the means of production is also familiar. Their consciousness of social place in the medical order, whether undesired or accepted, is not to be confused with class consciousness. Raymond Williams suggested (1977, 80) that the economic structure of society — Marx's sum of production relations (the foundation or base) and social institutions, forms of consciousness and political and cultural practices (the superstructure) — were not intended to be enclosed and abstract categories but a metaphorical association conveying 'the indissoluble connections between material production, political and cultural institutions and activity, and consciousness'. Even so, the determinative form of the base and superstructure link must suggest that consciousness is derivative. Then one puts aside subjective meanings (as, essentially, false consciousness) and searches, as Willis did, for the downwards operating forces that settle the occupational lot.

Bearing this in mind, whether the Indian caste system is an extreme version of class formation or of status grouping, or whether it has any cross-cultural application, is not to the point. Orthodox medical associations have isolated chiropractic, osteopathy and traditional acupuncture and have acted to check occupational mobility. All those concerned are well aware that material interests are at stake and they act to preserve them in a competitive situation. At the same time, segregation is enabled by deep-seated convictions about practitioner insufficiency and danger. These convictions are expressed by individuals and through them: the faceless writers of the AMA's 1992 paper on chiropractic both framed and represented an associational lore. People enact an order but they do so collectively.

The valuative idioms in which participants express their certitudes about the existence of objective occupational features ought not to be left aside or boiled down to epiphenomena by the use of structural typologies. To apprehend the occupational disposition, we pay heed to the entangled meanings that their own and other medicines have for those who work in them. That has been the endeavour in this study. In short, the organised divisions of healing work and the systematic ideations of occupational purpose give rise to and sustain each other. Another way of appreciating the coherence of health occupations and the divisions between them will be considered in the next section.

THE MAINTENANCE OF PLACE

When Gluckman (1956, 157) observed relations between the Zulus and whites, he thought at first that the opposition and hostility between them were absolute. Then he became increasingly aware of a large amount of co-operative activity. His conclusion was that 'conflicts in one set of relationships lead to the establishment of cohesion in a wider set of relationships' (p.164). The effect was realised within and through long-standing disputes, ambiguities, shifting intersections of interest and shared (though not equal) social and economic relations.

While coherence grew out of division, no amount of adjustment redressed the fundamental cleavage of the colour bar, as Gluckmann also noted (p. 163). We have seen that alternative health occupations continue to be kept apart. Their exclusion from the principal health agencies and services of the state measures the distance between them and other medicines.

Many alternative practitioners see each advance as at once a defeat of established opposition and a portent of eventual acceptance into the medical family. Others are less sanguine. American chiropractors were overjoyed at the successful result of a Supreme Court action provoked by established medical attempts to put them out of business (called the Wilk case).[1] Did that open the door to a new era? The dean of the chiropractic and osteopathy school was pessimistic. He told me:

> After the Wilk case, medicine decided to use another tactic. Instead of speaking out against chiropractic they have decided to block chiropractic in any way they can. I would do the same myself if I were them. It's my chiropractic paranoia speaking, maybe, but I think they will do anything to poison the well. There is no love lost still . . . It looks to me that things are getting worse, not better.

Later events, such as the AMA's publication of its attack on chiropractic (1992) and remarks addressed to doctors by one of its senior executives, made clear that medical association opposition to alternatives (and chiropractic was still labelled as such) was heating up.[2] Nevertheless, the dean continued to look for an accommodation. What incumbents say about their own and other health worker groups is guided by their expectation that the health occupations will be disposed, eventually, in a comprehensive array. The existence of a system, whether called the health care team or some other name, is supposed by the very occurrence of conflicts over due station in it. According to received wisdom, there is a prefigured health care order which implies that occupational placements will be settled according to it.

To talk about a health care system is to presume the existence of a totality of discrete parts. Patient care establishes the several purposes of the occupations — their division in the work of healing. They derive their content from varieties of sickness, for health workers assemble before the pathogenic sites. Through the appearance of its disorders, the body indicates occupational compartments.

While groups might be constituted by disease, they are aligned to each other in analogical response to the good body. Its ideal functioning suggests harmony, self-containment and interdependence. Therefore healing work is a graded unity, annexed to the interests of the organism and sharing its imperatives. In this manner of thinking, the condition for admission to the health care system is that an occupation becomes recognised by others as having an organic part. An alliance of health care organisation and biological order moves the authorised constituents towards destined states of occupational grace. The status of health profession is a vocational apotheosis. As a thing in itself, each profession has a nature that settles its identity and a function that determines its relations. Thus, the definition of an occupation generates a classification of the work lying outside as well as inside its range.

If the body provides this inner logic for the constitution and disposition of medical forces, then it also defines baneful interlopers. The irregular practitioners fuse with disorder itself. A doctor using chemotherapy loses the heroic battle against a patient's cancer but an alternative practitioner using herbs, manipulation or needles is culpably implicated in the death. In the pervasive warfare metaphor, only certified personnel have access to the medical armamentarium and only weapons in good standing are kept there.

The body and established occupations act vigorously to deal with morbid influences. A *Medical Journal of Australia* article (Donnelly et al., 1985, 539-540) comparing the utilisation of orthodox and other medicines began: 'There is much concern about the increasing popularity of alternative medicine, because of its pernicious effects on society and individual patients'. So far as many regular practitioners are concerned, there are two classes of health occupation: those, including their own, based in reason through the application of science and those pathological others that are irredeemably stained by falsehoods. Betwixt are the patients who, from the orthodox standpoint, mistakenly attribute their getting better (and often they only think they are better, sometimes they are actually worse) to the pseudoscience of the alternatives.

As they are scientifically unsound, the alternatives can not be efficacious. If evidence suggests that they are, then there has to be something wrong with the evidence. A chiropractic teacher attended a meeting where a rheumatologist said about a British report indicating substantial benefits from chiropractic treatment that 'they must have fudged their data'. Or if it is difficult to dismiss evidence of success on methodological or other grounds then the evidence is reinterpreted in a scientific idiom: an appropriate (that is, scientifically acceptable) explanation may not be readily available but it is just a matter of waiting for its eventual discovery. In this sense, science, like religion, embraces all.

The biological regulation of the health care system defines the sources of disorder, not only the external antagonists but also the internal disharmonies that weaken the resistant capacity of the occupational body. That is as true of established medicine as it is of the alternatives. On taking office, a new president of the Australian Medical Association was reported as having 'called for a closing of ranks within the association to prevent those outside from exploiting internal dissension to the detriment of the whole profession'. He said that without internal organisation 'we have chaos — we are defeated by anyone who wants to run us over'. He was 'emphatic that no one should be given an opportunity to use internal dissension to work against the association'.[3]

The division in health care, as many alternative practitioners see it, results from orthodox medical antipathy rather than from anything they say or do. Yet they make the same criticisms of each other. The alternatives, like the orthodox, argue about relations in terms of occupational substances. They also draw convictions about curative powers and privileged access from their special knowledge of and association with the body.

On obtaining some recognition, occupational associations sought to preserve the extant order, at least insofar as those considered to be inferior were concerned. The ACA expressed increasing concern to the Victorian health minister over:

> an apparent dramatic increase in the practice of manipulation by unregistered persons with no or little education in the discipline. The Association is particularly concerned over patient safety since the medical literature is replete of examples of patient injury from the use of manipulation by untrained persons.[4]

Having spoken of the duration and quality of chiropractic and osteopathy education at Phillip and of the insufficiency of the education available for masseurs and natural therapists, the ACA went on to propose the inclusion of practice limitations in the registration act. Their effect was to ban the use of manipulation by groups other than chiropractors and osteopaths and 'those persons with adequate training in other professions exempted from the Act, i.e. medical practitioners and physiotherapists'. The proposal, and the arguments for it, were similar to those made earlier to government about chiropractic and osteopathy by established medical and physiotherapy organisations.

The longstanding tendency of clinicians is, Kleinman noted (1980, 33), to treat healing as a totally independent, timeless, culture-free process. Medical organisations follow suit. The healing professions are considered to be natural things whose inherent characters are drawn from their organic relation. This is the believed order, in which work obtains its singularity by way of abnormal and normal bodily activity.

Medicines are often so built about the abstraction of biochemical and physiological operations that the social impress on bodily conceptions goes unremarked. The body, and the medical order along with it, are isolated in a literal metaphor. But Kleinman (1986: 193), using a cross-cultural perspective, suggested that the body was to be construed 'as a social, not a personal domain'. Attractive as this approach is, the medicines can be transported into another region: the organism might so far become an embodied social construction that disease nearly evaporates as a fact of nature and is replaced by a sociological category. In arguing against making a sharp distinction between disease as a biological disturbance and illness as a cultural phenomenon, Turner (1984, 208-209) considered the former to be a system of signs that could be read in various ways, with biology as a 'limiting horizon'.

This inversion could be supported by the argument that sociology, like alternative medicines themselves, was a dialectical counter to received views. Mary Douglas (1979, 122) suggested :

> Just as it is true that everything symbolises the body, so it is equally true (and all the more so for that reason) that the body symbolises everything else. Out of this symbolism, which in fold upon fold of interior meaning leads back to the experience of the self with its body, the sociologist is justified in trying to work in the other direction to draw out some of the layers of insight about the self's experience in society.

Bodies are territories with beginnings and ends but medical rights to them are disputed precisely because their containment holds endless prospects and uncertainties. Wittgenstein said the philosopher's treatment of a question was like the treatment of an illness (1988 I, §254). In answer to questions about bodily failings, the healers, like philosophers, respond with systems of knowing and treating which establish their own limits and move beyond them in claimancy. By taking their order in the figure of the body, the medicines will go on in an unceasing contention that is set by the terms for its disorders. It is a form of life: the enemies are within and without.

Notes

1. Wilk and four other chiropractors alleged that the American Medical Association and other groups had conspired to: monopolise health services; restrain chiropractors from competing with them; and isolate and eliminate chiropractors. The court found that there had been a restraint of trade. See the account in Wardwell (1992, ch. 8).
2. Wilkins, P. (Federal Assistant Secretary General of the AMA) 'Time to confront "alternative" therapies', *Australian Medicine*, 5, 7 (19 April 1993), p. 22. Wilkins said 'Most Australian doctors are well aware of the existence of "alternative" therapists and of the inroads they have made into conventional medical practice'. He went on to complain about successful public relations activities, false remedies and claims to treat conditions. 'Why doesn't someone/anyone do something/anything to curtail the activities of these groups?', he asked. He then said: 'the AMA would like to see doctors make more complaints to health departments and registration boards, and to ask their specialist and professional associations to protest about outlandish claims'.
3. Phillips, B., reported in 'After the Turmoil, a Closing of Ranks', *Medical Practice* 79, (6 June 1988) pp. 1-2.
4. Hylands, A., (Executive Secretary, ACA, Vic. branch), to Hogg, C., (Minister for Health), 1 August 1989, SCO files.

BIBLIOGRAPHY
(Where later editions and translations are cited,
first publication dates are given in square brackets after titles.)

Abbott, A. 1981, 'Status and Status Strain in the Professions', *American Journal of Sociology*, vol. 86, no. 4, pp. 819-833.

Abbott, A. 1988, *The System of Professions: An Essay on the Division of Expert Labor*, Chicago, University of Chicago Press.

AESO, 1987, 'An Evaluation of the Findings of the Victorian Social Development Committee', *Australian Journal of Traditional Chinese Medicine*, vol. 3, no. 2, pp. 21-25.

Albon, A. 1988, 'The wave theory of acupuncture', *Australian Journal of Traditional Chinese Medicine*, vol. 4, no. 2, pp. 20-35; vol. 4, no. 3, pp. 27-31.

Allport, G. 1958, *The Nature of Prejudice*, New York, Doubleday Anchor.

Althusser, L. 1977, *For Marx*, [1966], London, NLB.

AMA, 1992, *Chiropractic in Australia*, Australian Medical Association.

Anderson, R. 1981, 'Medicine, Chiropractic and Caste', *Anthropological Quarterly*, vol. 54, no. 3, pp. 157-165.

Antoni, C. 1962, *From History to Sociology: The Transition in German Historical Thinking*, [1940], London, Merlin Press.

Austin, J. 1962, *Sense and Sensibilia*, Oxford, University Press.

Baer, H. 1984, 'The Drive for Professionalization in British Osteopathy', *Social Science and Medicine*, vol. 19, no. 7, pp. 717-725.

Baer, H. 1987, 'The divergent evolution of osteopathy in America and Britain', *Research in the Sociology of Health Care*, vol. 5, pp. 63-99.

Banks, J. 1972, *The Sociology of Social Movements*, London, Macmillan.

Becker, H. P. 1932, 'Processes of secularisation: an ideal-typical analysis with special reference to personality change as affected by population movement', *Sociological Review*, vol. 24, pp. 138-154; pp. 266-287.

Becker, H. P. 1956, *Man in Reciprocity: Introductory Lectures on Culture, Society and Personality*, Westport (Conn.), Greenwood Press.

Becker, H. S. 1963, *Outsiders: Studies in the Sociology of Deviance*, New York, The Free Press/Macmillan.

Becker, H. S., Geer, B., Hughes, E. and Strauss, A. 1961, *Boys in White*, New York, Transaction Books.

Beckford, J. A. 1985, *Cult Controversies: the societal response to new religious movements*, London, Tavistock.

Ben-David, J. 1963-1964, 'Professions in the class system of present-day societies', *Current Sociology*, vol. 12, no. 3, pp. 247-330.

Berle, C. 1993, 'Legal opinion on W.A. case', *Australian Journal of Acupuncture*, vol. 20, p. 64.

Bernstein, B. 1973, 'On classification and framing of educational knowledge', in *Class, Codes and Control*, vol. 1: Theoretical Studies towards a Sociology of Language, St Albans, Paladin, pp. 227-278.

Bernstein, B. 1977, 'Class and pedagogies: visible and invisible', in *Class, Codes and Control*, vol. 3: Towards a Theory of Educational Transmissions, rev. edn., London, Routledge & Kegan Paul, pp. 116-156.

Berreman, G. 1960, 'Caste in India and the United States', *American Journal of Sociology*, vol. 66, no. 2, pp. 120-127.

Berreman, G. 1967, 'Stratification, pluralism and interaction: a comparative analysis of caste', in de Reuck, A. and Knight, J. (eds), *Caste and Race: Comparative Approaches*, London, Ciba Foundation/J. & A. Churchill, pp. 45-73.

Bloch, R. 1987, 'Methodology in clinical back pain trials', *Spine*, vol. 12, no. 5, pp. 430-432.

Bolton, S. 1959, A Study Affecting Chiropractic in Australia, ChD thesis, Davenport, Palmer College of Chiropractic.

Boyle, R. 1966, *Robert Boyle on Natural Philosophy*, Boas Hall, M. (ed.), Bloomington, Indiana University Press.

Braverman, H. 1974, *Labor and Monopoly Capitalism: The Degradation of Work in the Twentieth Century*, New York, Monthly Review Press.

Bromley, I. 1987, Editorial: 'The question of quality', *Physiotherapy Practice*, vol. 3, no. 4, p. 153.

Bryce, M.(ed.) 1987, *Pictorial History of the School of Chiropractic now at Phillip Institute of Technology*, Bundoora, Chiropractic Alumni Association, Phillip Institute of Technology.

CAA, 1993, *Chiropractors Fight Back: The Response to the Australian Medical Association's Position Paper 'Chiropractic in Australia'*, Faulconbridge, Chiropractors' Association of Australia (National) Limited.

Campbell, S. 1983, The Rise and Legitimation of Chiropractic: A Study of Professionalisation, MA thesis, Armidale, University of New England.

Campbell, S., Dillon, J. and Polus, B. 1982, 'Chiropractic in Australia: its development and legitimation', *Journal of the Australian Chiropractors' Association*, vol. 12, no. 4, pp. 21-30.

Cant, S. and Calnan, M. 1991, 'On the margins of the medical marketplace? An exploratory study of alternative practitioners' perceptions', *Sociology of Health and Illness*, vol. 13, no. 1, pp. 39-57.

Capra, F. 1976, *Tao of Physics: An Exploration of the Parallels between Modern Physics and Eastern Mysticism*, London, Fontana.

Charlton, K. 1986, 'The nature and environment of knowledge production, chiropractic theory and future progress', *Journal of the Australian Chiropractors' Association*, vol. 17, no. 2, pp. 46-48.

Charlton, K. 1987, 'Data and dogma: the use and abuse of information', *Journal of the Australian Chiropractors' Association*, vol. 16, no. 3, pp. 95-98.

Chinese Medical Classics, 1979, *The NEI CHING (Su Wen and Ling Shu) and NAN CHING*, Washington, Occidental Institute of Chinese Studies Alumni Association.

Cohn, N. 1970, *The Pursuit of the Millennium. Revolutionary Millenarians and Mystical Anarchists in the Middle Ages*, [1957], 3rd. edn., London, Paladin.

Collingwood, R. 1963, *The Idea of History* [1946], Oxford, University Press.

Coulter, I. 1983, 'Chiropractic observed: thirty years of changing sociological perspectives', *Chiropractic History*, vol. 3, no. 1, pp. 43-48.

Coulter, I. 1989, 'Chiropractic utilization: a statistical analysis', *American Journal of Chiropractic Medicine*, vol. 2, no. 1, pp. 13-21.

Cowie, J. and Roebuck, J. 1975, *An Ethnography of a Chiropractic Clinic: Definitions of a Deviant Situation*, New York, The Free Press/Macmillan.

Cyriax, J. 1973, Letter to the Editor: 'Registration of chiropractors', *Medical Journal of Australia*, vol. 1, no. 23, p. 1165.

De Vos, G. 1967, Discussion: 'Analogues and homologues of caste systems', in de Reuck, A. and Knight, J. (eds), *Caste and Race: Comparative Approaches*, London, Ciba Foundation/J. & A. Churchill, pp. 74-91.

Dix, N. 1985, Letter to the Editor: 'The practice of acupuncture', *Australian Journal of Physiotherapy*, vol. 31, no. 5, p. 208.

Dixon, J. (Chairperson) 1986, Parliament of Victoria, Social Development Committee: *Inquiry Into Alternative Medicine and the Health Food Industry*, 2 vols, Melbourne, Government Printer.

Doherty, R. (Chairman) 1988, Committee of Inquiry into Medical Education and Medical Workforce: *Australian Medical Education and Workforce into the 21st Century*, Canberra, Australian Government Publishing Service.

Dollard, J. 1957, *Caste and Class in a Southern Town*, [1937], 3rd edn., New York, Doubleday Anchor.

Donahue, J. 1986, 'D. D. Palmer and innate intelligence: development, division and derision', *Chiropractic History*, vol. 6, pp. 31-36.

Donnelly, J., Spykerboer, E. and Thong, Y. 1985, 'Are patients who use alternative medicine dissatisfied with orthodox medicine?', *Medical Journal of Australia*, vol. 142, no. 10, pp. 539-541.

Douglas, M. 1979, *Purity and Danger: An Analysis of the Concepts of Pollution and Taboo*, [1966], London, Routledge and Kegan Paul.

Douglas, M. 1973, *Natural Symbols*, Harmondsworth, Penguin.

Douglas, M. 1978, *Cultural Bias*, Occasional Paper no. 35, Royal Anthropological Institute of Great Britain and Ireland.

Dumont, L. 1967, 'Caste: a phenomenon of social structure or an aspect of Indian culture?', in de Reuck, A. and Knight, J. (eds), *Caste and Race: Comparative Approaches*, London, Ciba Foundation/J. & A. Churchill, pp. 28-38.

Dumont, L. 1972, *Homo Hierarchicus: The Caste System and its Implications* [1966], London, Paladin.

Durkheim, E. 1964, *The Division of Labour in Society*, [1893], New York, The Free Press.

Durkheim, E. 1982, *The Rules of Sociological Method: And selected texts on sociology and its method*, [1895], London, Macmillan.

Durkheim, E. and Mauss, M. 1969, *Primitive Classification*, [1903], 2nd edn., London, Cohen & West.

Erikson, K. 1966, *Wayward Puritans: A Study in the Sociology of Deviance*, New York, John Wiley & Sons.

Etzioni, A. 1966, *Studies in Social Change*, New York, Holt, Rinehart and Winston.

Flew, A. 1985, *Thinking about Social Thinking: The Philosophy of the Social Sciences*, Oxford, Basil Blackwell.

Foucault, M. 1973, *The Order of Things: An Archaeology of the Human Sciences*, [1966], New York, Vintage Books.

Foucault, M. 1976, *The Birth of the Clinic*, [1963], London, Tavistock.

Foucault, M. 1989, *Foucault Live (Interviews, 1966-84)*, Lotringer, S. (ed.), New York, Semiotext(e).

Fraser, P. 1990, 'Two scientific frameworks in acupuncture research. A review for the benefit of the Academic Board, La Trobe University, Melbourne', *Australian Journal of Traditional Chinese Medicine*, vol. 5, no. 2, pp. 5-10.

Frazer, J. 1911, *The Magic Art and the Evolution of Kings*, 3rd. ed., vol. 1 (Part 1 of *The Golden Bough: A Study of Magic and Religion*), [1890], London, Macmillan.

Freidson, E. 1970, *Professional Dominance: The Social Structure of Medical Care*, New York, Atherton Press.

Freidson, E. 1988a, *Profession of Medicine: A Study of the Sociology of Applied Knowledge* [1970], Chicago, University of Chicago Press.

Freidson, E. 1988b, *Professional Powers: A Study of the Institutionalization of Formal Knowledge*, Chicago, University of Chicago Press.

Galley, P. 1976, 'Patient referral and physiotherapy', *Australian Journal of Physiotherapy*, vol. 22, no. 3, pp. 117-120.

van Gennep, A. 1960, *The Rites of Passage*, [1908], Chicago, University of Chicago Press.

Gevitz, N. 1982, *The D.O.'s. Osteopathic Medicine in America*, Baltimore, Johns Hopkins University Press.

Gevitz, N. 1988, 'Osteopathic medicine: from deviance to difference', in Gevitz, N. (ed.) *Other Healers: Unorthodox Medicine in America*, Baltimore, Johns Hopkins University Press.

Gibbons, R. 1976, 'Chiropractic history: lost, strayed or stolen', *ACA Journal of Chiropractic*, vol. 13, no. 1, pp. 18-24.

Gibbons, R. 1978, 'Chiropractic history: turbulence and triumph the survival of a profession', in Dzaman, F. (ed.), *Who's Who in Chiropractic International 1976-1978*, Littleton, Chiropractic International Publishing, pp. 139-148.

Gibbons, R. 1980a, 'The rise of the chiropractic educational establishment 1897-1980', in Dzaman, F. (ed.), *Who's Who in Chiropractic International*, 2nd. edn., Littleton, Chiropractic International Publishing, pp. 339-352.

Gibbons, R. 1980b, 'The evolution of chiropractic: medical and social protest in America', in: Haldeman, S. (ed.), *Modern Developments in the Principles and Practice of Chiropractic*, New York, Appleton-Century-Crofts, pp. 3-24.

Glaser, B. and Strauss, A. 1971, *Status Passage*, London, Routledge & Kegan Paul.

Gluckman, M. 1956, *Custom and Conflict in Africa*, Oxford, Basil Blackwell

Gluckman, M. 1962, 'Les Rites de Passage', in Gluckman, M. (ed.), *Essays on the Ritual of Social Relations*, Manchester, University Press, pp. 1-52.

Godwin, W. 1976, *Enquiry Concerning Political Justice*, [1798], Harmondsworth, Penguin.

Guthrie, H. (Chairman) 1961, Honorary Royal Commission appointed to enquire into the provisions of the Natural Therapists Bill: *Report*, Perth, Government Printer.

Hahnemann, S. 1988, *Organon of Medicine*, [1810-1842], 6th edn., New Delhi, B. Jain Publishers.

Hawkins, P. and O'Neill, A. 1990, *Osteopathy in Australia*, Bundoora, Phillip Institute of Technology Press.

Hill, M. 1973, *A Sociology of Religion*, London, Heinemann.

Hill, M. 1992, 'New Zealand's cultic milieu: individualism and the logic of consumerism', in Wilson, B. (ed.), *Religion: Contemporary Issues – The All Souls Seminars in the Sociology of Religion*, London, Bellew Publishing.

Hill, M. 1993, 'Ennobled savages: New Zealand's manipulationist milieu', in Barker, E., Beckford, J. A. and Dobbelaere, K. (eds), *Secularization, Rationalism and Sectarianism: essays in honour of Bryan R. Wilson*, Oxford, Clarendon, pp. 145-165.

Himes, H. 1968/1969, 'The challenge of our future', *Digest of Chiropractic Economics* (a) July/August 1968, pp. 18-21; (b) September/October 1968, pp. 28-30; (c) January/Febuary 1969, pp. 24-26; (d) September/October 1969, pp. 20-23.

Hobbes, T. 1985, *Leviathan*, [1651], Harmondsworth, Penguin.

Hobsbawm, E. 1965, *Primitive Rebels: Studies in Archaic Forms of Social Movement in the 19th and 20th Centuries*, [1959], New York, W. W. Norton.

Hulme, T. 1960, *Speculations*, [1924], London, Routledge & Kegan Paul.

Illich, I. 1975, *Medical Nemesis: The Expropriation of Health*, London, Calder & Boyars.

Illich, I. 1977, 'Disabling Professions', in Illich, I., Zola, I., McKnight, J., Caplan, J. and Shaiken, H., *Disabling Professions*, London, Marion Boyars, pp. 11-39.

Jamison, J. 1985, 'Selection of a career in chiropractic', *Journal of the Australian Chiropractors' Association*, vol. 15, no. 1, pp. 32-34.

Jamous, J. and Peloille, B. 1970, 'Professions or Self Perpetuating Systems? Changes in the French University Hospital System', in Jackson, J. (ed.), *Professions and Professionalisation*, Cambridge, University Press, pp. 102-152.

Kaptchuk, T. 1983, *Chinese Medicine: The Web that has no Weaver*, London, Rider.

Kaufman, M. 1971, *Homeopathy in America*, Baltimore, Johns Hopkins University Press.

Kelner, M., Hall, O. and Coulter, I. 1980, *Chiropractors: Do They Help?*, Toronto, Fitzhenry & Whiteside.

Klegon, D. 1978, 'The sociology of the professions: an emerging perspective', *Sociology of Work and Occupations*, vol. 5, no. 259-283.

Kleinman, A. 1980, *Patients and Healers in the Context of Culture*, Berkeley, University of California Press.

Kleinman, A. 1986, *Social Origins of Distress and Disease: Depression, Neurasthenia, and Pain in Modern China*, New Haven, Yale University Press.

Kuhn, T. 1970, *The Structure of Scientific Revolutions*, [1962], 2nd. edn., International Encyclopedia of Unified Science, vol. 2, no.2 (Chicago, University of Chicago Press).

Layton, R. (Chairperson) 1986, Medicare Benefits Review Committee: *Second Report*, Canberra, Australian Government Publishing Service.

Lines, D. 1989a, 'Chiropractic in the 21st century: the past, the present and the future, Part 1: the past to the present', *Journal of the Australian Chiropractors' Association*, vol. 19, no. 1, pp. 29-33.

Lines, D. 1989b, 'Chiropractic in the 21st century: the past, the present and the future Part 2: the future: strategies for survival, growth and development', *Journal of the Australian Chiropractors' Association*, vol. 19, no. 2, pp. 49-54.

Lines, D. 1989c, 'Admissions criteria for selection of applicants for the B.App.Sc. (Chiropractic) at Phillip Institute of Technology: past practices and future recommendations', *Journal of the Australian Chiropractors' Association*, vol. 19, no. 4, pp. 142-148.

Lines, D. 1990, 'Reflections and looking ahead to the future', *Chiropractic Alumni Association News*, vol. 7, no. 5, pp. 20-21.

Liston, C. 1985, 'The use of acupuncture by physiotherapists', *Australian Journal of Physiotherapy*, vol. 31, no. 4, pp. 161-167.

Loy, J. (Chairman) 1990, Working Party on the Role and Requirements for Acupuncture Education: *Report*, Canberra, National Health and Medical Research Council.

Lu Gwei-Djen and Needham, J. 1980, *Celestial Lancets. A History and Rationale of Acupuncture and Moxa*, Cambridge, University Press.

McCorkle, T. 1961, 'Chiropractic: a deviant theory of disease and treatment in contemporary western culture', *Human Organization*, vol. 20, pp. 20-23.

McKenzie, R. 1989, 'A perspective on manipulative therapy', *Physiotherapy*, vol. 75, no. 8, pp. 440-444.

McLeod, J., Sainsbury, M. and Joseph, D. 1974, *Acupuncture: A Report to the National Health and Medical Research Council*, Canberra, Australian Government Publishing Service.

Malcolm, J. 1977, 'Socialisation in the medical school — the hidden curriculum', paper for the 5th Annual Conference of the Australasian and New Zealand Association for Medical Education, 27 August.

Malinowski, B. 1974, 'Magic, science and religion', [1925], in: *Magic, Science and Religion and Other Essays*, London, Souvenir Press.

Marx, K. 1954, *Capital: A Critique of Political Economy*, [1867-1883], Moscow, Progress Publishers.

Miles-Tapping, C. 1985, 'Physiotherapy and medicine: dominance and control?', *Physiotherapy Canada*, vol. 37, no. 5, pp. 289-293.

Mills, T. 1967, *The Sociology of Small Groups*, Englewood Cliffs, Prentice-Hall.

Munro-Ashman, J. and Quail, A. 1979, *Traditional Medicine and Acupuncture in China: A three month study tour Sept.-Nov. 1977*, Canberra, Department of Health and National Health and Medical Research Council.

Murthy, J. and Naidu, K. 1988, 'Aneurysm of the cervical internal carotid artery following chiropractic manipulation', *Journal of Neurology Neurophysiology and Psychiatry*, vol. 51, no. 9, pp. 1237-1238.

Myerhoff, B. 1977, 'We don't wrap herring in a printed page: fusion, fictions and continuity in secular ritual', in Moore, S. and Myerhoff, B. (eds), *Secular Ritual*, Assen/Amsterdam, Van Gorcum, pp. 199-224.

Needham, J. 1954-1988, *Science and Civilization in China*, Cambridge University Press. V. 2 1962, *History of Scientific Thought*; (with Lu Gwei-Djen) V. 6, 1980 (part), *Celestial Lancets: A History and Rationale of Acupuncture and Moxa*.

Needham, J. 1970, 'Medicine and Chinese culture', [1966], in Needham, J. *Clerks and Craftsmen in China and the West: Lectures and addresses on the history of science and technology*, Cambridge, University Press.

Nicholls, P. 1988, *Homoeopathy and the Medical Profession*, London, Croom Helm.

Nisbet, R. 1969, *Social Change and History*, Oxford, University Press.

O'Neill, A. 1989, 'The luetic neighbour', *Australian Educational Researcher*, vol 16, no.2, pp. 45-56.

O'Neill, A. 1990, 'Sharpening the front end: investigating acupuncture', *Australian Journal of Acupuncture*, vol. 14, pp. 38-54.

O'Neill, A. 1991a, 'The double edged sword: more about investigating acupuncture', *Australian Journal of Acupuncture*, vol. 15, pp. 39-44.

O'Neill, A. 1991b, *Enemies Within and Without: Educating Chiropractors, Osteopaths and Traditional Acupuncturists*, Ph. D. thesis, Armidale, University of New England.

Palmer, B. J. 1906-1910, *The Science of Chiropractic*, Davenport, The Palmer School of Chiropractic.

Palmer, B. J. 1939, *The Electroencephaloneuromentimpograph*, Davenport, Palmer School of Chiropractic.

Palmer, B. J. n.d.?1959, *Shall Chiropractic Survive?*, Davenport, Palmer School of Chiropractic.

Palmer, B. J. 1979, *Up From Below The Bottom*, [1950], 2nd. edn., Spartanburg, Sherman College of Straight Chiropractic.

Palmer, D. D. 1910, *The Chiropractor's Adjuster: Textbook of the Science, Art and Philosophy of Chiropractic*, Portland, Portland Printing House (facsimile edition).

Paracelsus 1990, 'Das Buch Paragranum', [1529-30], in *Paracelsus: Essential Readings*, Wellingborough, Crucible.

Parkin, F. 1974, 'Strategies of social closure in class formation', in Parkin, F. (ed.), *The Social Analysis of Class Structure*, London, Tavistock, pp. 1-18.

Parkin, F. 1979, *Marxism and Class Theory: A Bourgeois Critique*, London, Tavistock.

Partridge, C. 1987, 'Evaluation of the efficacy of ultrasound', *Physiotherapy*, vol. 73, no. 4, pp. 46-48.

Passin, H. 1967, Discussion: 'A comparative approach to caste and race', in de Reuck, A. and Knight, J. (eds), *Caste and Race: Comparitive Approaches*, London, Ciba Foundation/J. & A. Churchill, pp. 327-332.

Popper, K. 1972, *Conjectures and Refutations: The Growth of Scientific Knowledge*, [1963], 4th ed., London, Routledge & Kegan Paul.

Porkert, M. (with Ullman, C.) 1988, *Chinese Medicine*, New York, William Morrow.

Ransom, J. 1985, 'The origins of chiropractic physiological therapeutics: Howard, Forester and Schulze', *Chiropractic History*, vol. 4, no. 1, pp. 47-52.

Rayner, S. 1986, 'The politics of schism: routinisation and social control in the International Socialists/Socialist Workers' Party', in Law, J. (ed.), *Power, Action and Belief: A New Sociology of Knowledge?*, Sociological Review Monograph 32, London, Routledge & Kegan Paul, pp. 46-67.

Reiser, J. 1978, *Medicine and the Reign of Technology*, Cambridge, University Press.

Resnick, J. 1990, 'An open letter to acupuncturists', *Australian Journal of Acupuncture*, vol. 14, pp. 33-35.

Resnick, J. 1991, 'An open letter to acupuncturists # 2', *Australian Journal of Acupuncture*, vol. 15, pp. 35-36.

Resnick, J. 1993, 'Acupuncturists beware!', *Australian Journal of Acupuncture*, vol. 20, p. 63.

Robertson, R. 1972, *The Sociological Interpretation of Religion*, Oxford, Basil Blackwell.

Rose, H 1979, 'Hyper-Reflexivity – a new danger for the counter-movements', in Nowotny, H. and Rose, H. (eds), *Counter-Movements in the Sciences*, Dordrecht, Reidel, pp. 277-289.

Rosenthal, S. 1981, 'Marginal or mainstream: two studies of contemporary chiropractic', *Sociological Focus*, vol. 14, no. 4, pp. 271-285.

Roth, J. 1957, 'Ritual and magic in the control of contagion', *American Sociological Review*, vol. 22, no. 3, pp. 310-314.

Roth, J. 1977, *Health Purifiers and their Enemies*, New York, Prodist.

Salmon, J. 1984, 'Introduction', in Salmon, J. (ed.), *Alternative Medicines: Popular and Policy Perspectives*, New York, Tavistock, pp. 1-29.

Schumpeter, J. 1955, 'Social classes in an ethnically homogeneous environment', [1927], in Schumpeter, J., *Imperialism and Social Classes: Two Essays*, New York, Meridian Books, pp. 99-168.

Schwartz, B. 1985, *The World of Thought in Ancient China*, Cambridge (Mass.), Belknap Press/Harvard University Press.

Sheehan, M. (Consultant) 1985, *Report to the National Chiropractic Consultative Committee on a Review of Chiropractic Services*, Brisbane, Uniquest (University of Queensland).

Sontag, S. 1983, *Illness as Metaphor*, Harmondsworth, Penguin.

Sorel, G. 1961, *Reflections on Violence*, [1906/1908], New York, Collier.

Sportelli, L. 1989, 'The laying on of hands', *ACA Journal of Chiropractic*, vol. 26, no. 12, pp. 99-100.

Stephenson, R. 1948, *Chiropractic Textbook*, Davenport, Palmer School of Chiropractic.

Sternberg, D. 1969, Boys in Plight: A Case Study of Chiropractic Students Confronting a Medically-Oriented Society, PhD thesis, New York, New York University.

Still, A. 1897, *Autobiography*, Kirksville, Published by the Author.

Still, A. 1899, *Philosophy of Osteopathy*, Kirksville, Published by the Author

Still, A. 1902, *The Philosophy and Mechanical Principles of Osteopathy*, Kansas City, Hudson-Kimberley Publishing (Osteopathic Enterprise facsimile edition).

Still, A. 1908, *Autobiography*, 2nd edn., Kirksville, Published by the Author (Academy of Applied Osteopathy, facsimile edition).

Still, A. 1910, *Osteopathy. Research and Practice*, Kirksville, Published by the Author.

Taylor, R. 1979, *Medicine Out of Control: The Anatomy of a Malignant Technology*, Melbourne, Sun Books.

Terrett, A. 1986, 'The Genius of D.D. Palmer', *Journal of the Australian Chiropractors' Association*, vol. 16, no. 4, pp. 150-158.

Tönnies, F. 1957, *Community and Society*, [1887], East Lansing, Michigan State University Press.

Townsend, L. (Chairman) 1982, *Report to the Health Commission on Registration of Acupuncturists*, Melbourne, Victorian Health Advisory Council.

Troeltsch, E. 1931, *The Social Teachings of the Christian Churches*, [1911], 2 vols, London, George Allen and Unwin.

Turner, B. 1984, *The Body and Society*, Oxford, Basil Blackwell.

Twomey, L. 1983, 'The physiotherapist', *Medical Journal of Australia*, vol. 1, no. 9, pp. 422-424.

Twomey, L. and Cole, J. 1985, 'The changing face of Australian physiotherapy', *Physiotherapy Practice*, vol. 1, no. 2, pp. 77-85.

Unschuld, P. 1985, *Medicine in China: A History of Ideas*, Berkeley, University of California Press.

Unschuld, P. 1987, 'Traditional Chinese Medicine: Some Historical and Epistemological Reflections', *Social Science and Medicine*, vol. 24, no. 12, pp. 1023-1029.

Ward, H. (Chairman) 1975, Osteopathy, Chiropractic and Naturopathy Committee: *Report*, Melbourne, Government Printer.

Wardwell, W. 1952, 'A marginal professional role: the chiropractor', *Social Forces*, vol.30, pp. 339-348.

Wardwell, W. 1976, 'Orthodox and unorthodox practitioners: changing relationships and the future status of chiropractors', in Wallis, R. and Morley, P. (eds), *Marginal Medicine*, New York, Macmillan/Free Press, pp. 61-73.

Wardwell, W. 1980, 'The present and future role of the chiropractor', in Halderman, S. (ed.), *Modern developments in the principles and practice of chiropractic*, New York, Appleton-Century-Crofts, pp. 25-41.

Wardwell, W. 1988, 'Chiropractors: evolution to acceptance', in Gevitz, N. (ed.), *Other Healers: Unorthodox medicine in America*, Baltimore, Johns Hopkins University Press, pp. 157-191.

Wardwell, W. 1992, *Chiropractic: History and Evolution of a New Profession*, St Louis, Mosby Year Book.

Warner, W. Lloyd. 1936, 'American caste and class', *American Journal of Sociology*, vol. 42, no. 2, pp. 234-237.

Watts, A. 1972, *The Way of Zen*, [1957], Harmondsworth, Penguin.

Webb, E. (Chairman) 1977, Chiropractic, Osteopathy, Homoeopathy and Naturopathy Committee: *Report*, Canberra, Commonwealth Government Printer.

Weber, M. 1948, *From Max Weber. Essays in Sociology*, London, Routledge and Kegan Paul.

Weber, M. 1978, *Economy and Society*, [1914-1920], Berkeley, University of California Press.

Westerman, R. (Chairman) 1988, *Acupuncture: A NHMRC Working Party Report*, Canberra, National Health and Medical Research Council.

Westerman, R. (Chairman) 1989, *Acupuncture*, Canberra, National Health and Medical Research Council.

Whyte, W. 1984, *Learning From The Field: A Guide From Experience*, Beverly Hills, Sage.

Wiesner, D. 1983, Professionalization Under Domination: the Natural Therapies in Australia, PhD thesis, Sydney, University of New South Wales.

Wild, P. 1978, 'Social origins and ideology of chiropractors: an empirical study of the socialization of the chiropractic student', *Sociological Symposium*, vol. 22, pp. 33-54.

Williams, R. 1977, *Marxism and Literature*, Oxford, University Press.

Williamson, J., George, T., Simpson, D., Hannah, B. and Bradbury, E. 1986, 'Ultrasound in the treatment of ankle sprains', *Injury*, vol. 17, no. 3, pp. 176-178.

Willis, E. 1981, The Division of Labour in Health Care, PhD thesis, Clayton, Monash University.

Willis, E. 1983, rev. edn. 1989, *Medical Dominance*, Sydney, George Allen & Unwin.

Willis, E. 1989, 'Complementary healers', in Lupton, G. and Najman, J. (eds), *Sociology of Health and Illness Australian Readings*, Melbourne, Macmillan, pp. 259-279.

Wilson, B. R. 1973, *Magic and the Millennium: a sociological study of religious movements of protest among tribal and third-world peoples*, London, Heinemann.

Wittgenstein, L. 1988, *Philosophical Investigations*, [1953], 3rd edn., Oxford, Basil Blackwell.

INDEX
Compiled by Kerry Herbstreit

ANGLO-EUROPEAN COLLEGE OF CHIROPRACTIC

ANGLO-EUROPEAN COLLEGE OF CHIROPRACTIC